FIT
HAPPENS
... AT ANY AGE

D1548246

by MICHAEL S. PIERRON
Motivational Speaker
Triathlete,
Masters physique competitor and
Former Fat Guy!

Training
Nutrition
Time

(in the right balance)

www.DRMBIG.com

Caution:

Assess your health status and *consult your physician* before beginning any exercise program. *Fit Happens ... at any age* was written in a fun, fast-moving, informational format. It has been a 25-year research project – but is not intended as medical advice.

It will, however, help most people get into the best shape of their lives *and* potentially become their own personal trainers!

Fit Happens ... *at any age!*
Copyright © 2002 by Mike Pierron.
Printed and bound in the United States of America.
All rights reserved.

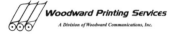
Woodward Printing Services
A Division of Woodward Communications, Inc.

Dedication

Every writer has a source of inspiration,

For me... it's Chelsea Hollrith.

She, along with her sister Ashley, were the first to call me
"Muscle Mike".

It is in Chelsea's cherished memory, that this book is dedicated.

Tam:
Great meeting you... as you know,
Fit Does Happen
By Choice
12/20/12
Muscle Mike

Special Thanks

Thanks also to… Mr. Cliff

A person I never met, but who helped get me through high school and college:

Mr. Cliff passed away at age 91 in 2001.

He was the creator of

"Cliff Notes"

as a way to help readers better understand fine literature.

I tried to provide my own brand of "Cliff Notes" for fitness, nutrition and motivational information. Here's hoping **Fit Happens** will help you, as much as Mr. Cliff helped me get through the many weeks of Shakespeare.

DREAM BIG!

"If one advances confidently in the direction of their dreams, and endeavors to live the life which they have imagined, they will meet a success unexpected in common hours."

- Henry David Thoreau

Life is dull to dull people.
Life is exciting to exciting people!

Table of Contents

Chapter 1

Dream Big and Get Fit

"Do not follow where the path leads, but go where there is no path and leave a trail."

- Grafton High School
Senior Motto 1981

"Progress is impossible without change."

- Walt Disney

"Make visible what, without you, might perhaps never have been seen."

- Robert Bresson,
French film director

"Every human is an artist. The dream of your life is to make beautiful art."

- don Miguel Ruiz,
Author

"Use your imagination not to scare yourself to death,
but to inspire yourself to life."

- Adele Brookman,
Psychotherapist

The Road Map to Fitness

As a consultant, if you asked me for the best driving route from Los Angeles to New York I'd recommend consulting a proven route – a map. Now let's say I've got the only map in the United States. What would it be worth to you?

Now, what if millions of people wanted the same map? Guess what, they do - and it's only $14.95. You are now holding the map to your fitness success in your hands. Here's hoping you follow the directions, and arrive at your destination on time.

*Good news: Just like traveling cross-country, you can start whenever you like, and arrive whenever you care, and even stop along the way to appreciate the beauty of the trip. But it's up to you to want to make the trip. Fit happens by choice, not by chance.

The trick is to make a personal commitment to yourself.
Never give up!
Never give in! And most importantly ...
Enjoy the journey!

"Most people fail, not because of lack of desire, but, because of lack of commitment."

- Vince Lombardi

The reason 97 percent of New Year's resolutions fail each year is because of lack of commitment.

Change the "I resolve to blah, blah, blah" to "*I commit, that I will follow the TNT system for the next 90 days in order to get the results I always knew were possible.*"

Hey, America, We're Getting Fatter!

A Journal of American Medical Association editorial that accompanies a story on the growing obesity problem among U.S. adults says many things are to blame:

- A plentiful supply of fattening foods (most fast food)

- Sedentary (non-active) lifestyles

- Cultural factors

- Genetics

For most of us, it boils down to this: *Eat too much, exercise too little.* Add to that a bit of old-fashioned laziness and you've got yourself a fat country.

Motivational message from a former fat guy… Results!

One of the toughest things about working out is getting started. Personally, I've begun a training program at least a dozen times. I've also quit a dozen times.

You are probably no different.

Maybe getting started, though, is the easy part. (Heck, we seem to do it every year.)

Instead it seems that sticking with it and making a lifestyle commitment seems to be our problem.

In an attempt to solve the mystery of "why do we quit?" I wrote this book. You see, I feel the answer that plagues most unfit people lies in one word … *results*! Meaning if you begin to see "positive results" in the mirror (not on the scale), you will then become more motivated to "stick with it!"

Thus, the why America quits question is answered because we (most of the time with an overemphasis on cardio, aerobics, kickboxing, etc.) will eventually plateau and cease to see visible results.

You hit the dreaded "fitness plateau."

Then, confused on what to do next … other than overtrain (thinking "more is better" and begin performing i.e., more exercise, more aerobics, more everything) … you eventually give up and settle for the body that fate dealt you. You do this by rationalizing "Well, this is how I am"!

Sound familiar … Oprah?

Happiness is a Choice!

Seven sure-fire ways to help people live happier, less-stressed lives:

1) Stop comparing yourself to others. It does nothing positive; it only distances you from people you truly care about.

2) Do the things you fear. Whenever you avoid dealing with something, ask yourself: "Why?" If it's because you fear failure, force yourself to try it. There are valuable lessons to be learned from *finally facing your fears*.

3) Break your routine. Try new ways of getting ready in the morning ... drive new roads to work ... create new strategies to organize your time. This will open up new ways of solving problems, and you'll begin to think more creatively, freeing yourself from what you thought was normal.

4) Rid yourself of anger. Channel your excess energy into an effective stress- reduction program – like exercise.

5) Ignore an insult. In doing so, it prevents you from being consumed by someone else's negative energy.

6) Learn to forgive. Don't let negative experiences hinder you from moving forward. Continue to fail forward.

7) Smile more. If you do all of the above, smiling will become a natural by-product. An added benefit: You'll scare the heck out of everyone around you!

(Life is a self-fulfilling prophecy. You can "think yourself happier" if you want to. Try it!)

Chapter 2

TNT Overview – Losing the Fat

What Do You Want to Be When You Grow Up?

For me it was ...

Age 3   Superman.

Age 7   President of the U.S.

Age 10 Professional athlete

Age 17 All-county/all-conference in baseball and basketball.

Age 18 Major League Baseball tryout with the Kansas City Royals. (Wasn't offered a contract ... not good enough!) .

Age 19 Hit .443 and was named all-league ... my last year in baseball.

Age 20 "Cut" for the second time trying out for the University of Wisconsin-Whitewater baseball team.

Age 20 One month later, became a Resident Assistant (R.A.) in Wells Hall (East) and was elected Vice President of the American Marketing Association the next semester.

The point:
Dreaming big and failing is OK.

The result:
After my first battle with depression, I set newer, higher, different goals.

The Turning Point of My Life

At 20, I was cut a second time from the University of Wisconsin-Whitewater baseball team tryouts. That day was the toughest of my life.

After much reflection (read: depression) I realized my goal of becoming the next Robin Yount was over …

I had to find a new goal, and quickly …

New goal: Become one of the most requested and respected motivational speakers in the world!

So, in answer to the question: "How long does it take to become an overnight success?"… about twenty years.

The end result ...

"Twenty years from now, you'll be
more disappointed by the things you
didn't do, than the ones you did."

- Mark Twain

Explore, discover, and dream ... BIG!

Character is what you build when times are tough.

Characteristics of Fit, Successful People:

Proactive
Creative
Open-minded
Assertive
Sensitive to time
Priority-based
Curious
Honest
Great listener
Eager to learn
Resourceful
Respected
Intuitive
Courageous
Focused
Helpful
Positive

Is this how you see yourself?

If not, you can change ... for the better.

E + A = R

Education + Attitude = Results

Success in reaching your fitness goals is based on sticking to a set of common sense principles that anyone can master.

You Can Do It!

Think: "If it's meant to be, it's up to me."

TNT Overview

Training
2-3 weight resistance workouts per week.

30-45 minutes per workout – tops!

Nutrition
Match your nutrition with your goals. Eat and drink more protein.
Eat smarter meals more often, and add plenty of water.

Time
Allow time and rest to work for you … not against you
Do not overtrain!

The Stress of Life

In his book, *The Stress of Life*, author Hans Selye defined stress as the rate of wear and tear on the body.

Resistance (strength) training is a type of stress. Although self-inflicted, it involves a more intense breakdown and destruction of muscle tissue than does everyday living.

How do you compensate for the breakdown of muscle tissue that occurs during a high-intensity workout? Rest, sleep, naps, proper nutrition, and time. When these key elements are added, the results are new muscle growth, a higher metabolism, and more efficient fat-burning.

Think:
• Weight training to stimulate muscle growth, and
• Nutrition/Diet to positively change body appearance (i.e. lose the fat)

Chapter 3
Weight Training For Life

Tales from the Gym

Susan has been taking a one-hour aerobics class three times per week for the past four years. She still carries extra fat – especially on her legs, hips and butt.

Before her 10-year class reunion, she stepped up her routine to six times per week. Only by doing that was she finally able to reduce her body fat and enjoy a lean figure for the event.

After the reunion, Susan went back to exercising only three times per week. Being thin just wasn't worth all that extra time in the gym. Within a couple of months, the fat was back. She figured that this was the way her body meant to be.

Fit Solution:

Three times a week is enough trips to the gym, as long as you do the correct exercises while you are there! Having traveled all over the world and no matter where I go, the "least fit" people in the gym are doing aerobics. **Cardiovascular exercises do not burn fat as efficiently as weight training.** More muscle means better fat burning 24 hours a day! – Muscle burns fat 24/7! Yes – that's even while you sleep. Susan's time would be better spent in the **result room** – (read: weight room.)

She can have her thin figure by weight training only three times per week for thirty minutes at a time. In fact, working out more often than that will almost always lead to over-training, if the intensity is high enough.

Reasons to Weight Train for Life

1) More muscle means better fat-burning ability. (Muscle burns fat 24/7.)

2) More muscle means a stronger immune system.

3) More muscle strengthens bones and lowers blood pressure.

4) Strength training increases your energy levels.

5) Strength training improves athletic performance.*

6) Strength training improves physical appearance. (Duh!)

7) Strength training improves balance, coordination and circulation.

8) Strength training helps relaxation and promotes a good night's sleep.

9) Strength training prevents bone loss as we age (osteoporosis).

10) Strength training increases self-confidence/self-esteem.**

*My Reason for beginning weight training at age 14
**The greatest benefit of a result-producing program like TNT.

Confusing Questions

Q. Can anyone, at any age, improve his or her level of fitness?
A. Yes!

Q. What is the single-best exercise?
A. The best exercise is a compound exercise requiring the entire body:
   1. Deadlifts - followed closely by
   2. Squats

Q. No, not a "weight-training exercise." I meant to ask ... What is the single best fat-burning exercise?
A. Deadlifts – followed closely by squats

Q. Well, I'm confused. I thought cardiovascular exercises, such as aerobics, are best for fat burning?!
A. Wrong! You asked about the single best exercise. Kick boxing, step aerobics, jogging, swimming, and bicycling all do, to varying degrees, burn calories. But when it comes to burning fat, nothing works as well as high-intensity weight training performed 2-3 times per week.

Q. What is TNT?
A. TNT is an exclusive training system developed for the time-starved, busy baby-boomer. It's the ideal combination of proper:
   Training
   Nutrition and
   Time

Effective Training, matching your Nutrition to your goals, and allowing Time:
1. For improvements to happen.
2. For your body to recuperate, rest, grow, and burn fat between work outs.

Q. What time of the day should I train?
A. Any time you can.

Q. No, I meant what is the best time of day to train in order to burn the most fat?
A. First thing in the morning on an empty stomach! Fact: You will burn two to three times more fat first thing in the morning on an empty stomach than at any other time of day.

(Hint: Read that again .... slowly. You will burn two to three times more fat first thing in the morning on an empty stomach as compared to any other time of the day. Wow!)

Q. Why?
A. You haven't eaten for nearly eight hours. When you exercise, most of what you burn will come from stored fat, which is used as energy to fuel your workout.

Keep in mind, that the order your body uses food for energy is ...

1. Simple carbohydrates (candy, simple sugars, fruits)
2. Complex carbohydrates (potatoes, rice)
3. Protein (fish, poultry, meat and eggs)
4. Fat (salmon, peanuts, avocados)

So, if you haven't eaten anything for eight hours, your body has *no choice* but to skip right to burning your *stored fat for energy*.

TNT Secret #1
Morning workouts burn the most fat!

Get It Right!

Deadlifts and squats burn the most fat!

Why: Large muscle groups – compound, multi-joint intense exercises.

Deadlifts train big muscles (hamstrings, glutes, thighs, etc.)

Women prefer "rounded, athletic-looking glutes" on men
(Men's Health, Nov. 2001)

**Men typically work hard to develop a strong chest,
while women prefer and notice an athletic butt.**

Commentary: "*Hello ... McFly! We're training the wrong stuff!*"

"If the blind lead the blind, both shall fall into the ditch"

- Matthew 15:14

Exercise:
The Key to Fat Control.

The best way to lose fat is by exercising off the excess (i.e., burn more calories than you take in). "First on, last off": Sounds like an accounting principle, but actually it's your body's natural fat storage system. For men, this means your problem areas are lower abs and lower back. For women, problem areas are hips, glutes, hamstrings and triceps. Both aerobics (i.e., using oxygen) and anaerobic exercises (i.e. high intensity weight training) burn calories. It's not how much you do that's important, it's how "intensely" you do it. If you can hold up your end of a conversation while working out, you're not burning as much fat as you could be.

Suggestion! Forget that fat-burning, range-thinking nonsense and merely raise your intensity level!

The biggest benefit of high-intensity weight training is that you burn calories both while exercising and when your body is at rest (the rest of the day). With every increase in muscle mass, you increase your fat-burning ability, both while you train and while you rest.

* Muscle burns fat 24/7!

Your Bathroom Scale

1. For best results, throw it away!

"It's not what you weigh, it's what you look like you weigh that counts."

Muscle weighs 2-3 times as much as fat.

Deadlifts:
The Best Fat-Burning Exercise

Deadlifts are so called because the end result is usually "death" by fatigue. Seriously, though, dead lifts are great for creating a rock solid foundation by strengthening your back, stabilizing your posture, developing your trunk muscles, and kick-starting your fat-burning potential.

Starting Position: I prefer "heavy dumbbells." Heavy is a relative term – they should allow you to perform 8-12 repetitions. Stand with the dumbbells almost touching your shins, feet flat on the floor and shoulder-width apart. Place your hands slightly wider than your shoulders, outside your knees. Keep your back flat, arms straight, shoulders over the bar, and head and eyes straight ahead.

The Exercise: Pull the dumbbells up by straightening your legs and moving your hips forward while raising your shoulders to a shrug position. Do not round your back during the lift – keep your back flat and strong! Throughout the dead lift, make sure that the dumbbells are close to your body, your feet are flat on the floor, and your arms are straight. As you raise the dumbbells over your knees, drive your hips forward and keep pulling up until your knees are under the bar. By now, your body should be almost vertical, your head straight and facing forward, your feet flat, your shoulders back, and your arms straight. Though you are using all your muscles to pull the bar up, your primary goal is to drive the weight up with your legs – primarily "pushing" with your heels. When you reach the top position of the dead lift, keep your legs straight and your body erect. Pause at the top of the move and then slowly lower the dumbbells, bending your legs. Squat down.

Breathing Technique: As with every exercise, breathe! During the dead lift, exhale through the upward motion and inhale during the downward motion.

Rep Cadence: "2, 3, 4" – 2 seconds on the positive portion, 3 seconds on a "static hold," and 4 seconds on the negative portion.

"Fitness success is a lot like wrestling a gorilla. You don't quit when you're tired – you quit when the gorilla is tired."

Don't Be Afraid Of an "F" Word! (Hint: Fear)

1. Fear of the result room. The result room is the weight room. The fine-tuning room is the cardio room. Don't be concerned with fine-tuning until the frame is repaired.

2. Failure is your friend. While exercising, try to reach the point of "momentary muscular failure." This is where you can't even do one more repetition in good form.

3. Future: KISS – Keep It Simple, Stupid, or

Knowledge   +

Intensity   +

Short Workouts   +

Sweat   =   Results.

Attitude makes the difference. Always has, always will.

Chapter 4

Ten Commandments of Fitness Success

After analyzing my own experiences (and training failures) and answering thousands of questions from people all over the world, I've identified TEN ESSENTIAL STEPS TO take your physique to the next level.

Ten Commandments of Fitness Success™

I. Take Responsibility. Take responsibility for becoming a "student" of your fitness success. Shorten your fitness learning curve by thinking **logically** about your training and nutrition.

II. Apply the Power of TNT to reach your fitness goals. Learn proper **Training**, match your **Nutrition** with your goals, and allow **Time** for it all to work.

III. Dream Big! Believe that getting in the best shape of your life is possible, regardless of your age.

IV. Develop the Action Habit and **Move**! Think priority management, effectiveness, and efficiency.

V. Invest in the Fitness Lifestyle. Understand exercise is a "two for one" special. For every one hour you exercise, it's proven, you gain an extra two hours of quality living.

VI. For Best Results ... Throw Away Your Scale! It doesn't matter how **much** you weigh, it matters how much you look like you weigh. *(Hint: Muscle weighs twice as much as fat)*

VII. Drink More Water. Strive to drink eight to ten glasses of pure water each day.

VIII. Become a Morning Person. You will burn two to three times more fat first thing in the morning on an empty stomach than any other time of the day!

IX. Think High-Intensity Training. Stick to basic, compound, exercises to burn the most fat, and add variety to enjoy each visit.

X. Have faith and be patient. More is not better. Better is better! Be efficient and intense with your training, but not long. Limit yourself to three weekly trips to the gym, on non-consecutive days – at the most. Guard against overtraining like the plague.

If it's meant to be, it's up to me.

Proven steps to improve your fitness level:
Examine/improve your nutritional choices and lifestyle.
Match your nutrition to your goals.
"Think" of self-help health care (i.e., take care of yourself)

When thinking about how much training you need ...

How much is too much?
It's not how much you do, but rather how you do it that matters most.

Guard against overtraining like the plague – it's not only negative, it's **counterproductive**.

"I will go anywhere as long as it's forward."
- David Livingston

Chapter 5
The 3-2-1 Priority System

Exercise Has No Negatives

None, whatsoever – unless you train too much (or too long)

There is a priority system of which exercises burn the most fat, which should be followed to yield the most effective results.

Ready ...

1. Deadlifts

2. Squats

3. Leg Presses

4. Back

5. Chest

6. Shoulders

7. Triceps and calves

8. Biceps

9. Abs

... In that order

Hint: Their order (sequence) is official. Start training the largest body parts first, when you're fresh, in order to burn the most calories/fat.

Tales from the Gym:

Danielle is a 30-year-old woman with a naturally thin physique. Even with her genetic advantage, the birth of her son two years ago left her with some very real figure flaws. Her stomach, and even her back are kind of loose and flabby. On her upcoming vacation, she is hoping to wear a bikini with pride. Because she doesn't have much time to get in shape, she decides to really focus on her worst problem area – the abs. She figures if her stomach is tight, she'll look good no matter what.

In order to really get those abs tight fast, she orders The Gut Buster. According to the infomercial, she will have a six-pack stomach in less than a month if she uses the Gut Buster for just 20 minutes per day. The price was right – only $49.95! What a deal!

"Gut Busters"
Why They Don't Work

Results. Proven results. That is what most people are looking for while watching a "Gut Buster" infomercial on late night TV.

The problem is "Gut Busters" don't work. Oh, you will likely strengthen your abdominal wall, but to finally see your abs, you need to *burn the fat off first!*

The best way to burn fat? High-intensity, short-duration, compound exercises like weight training, combined with a high-protein nutritional plan, complete with essential fatty acids.

As a performance improvement consultant' my goal is to inspire others to get results in the most efficient way possible.

That's not to say that hours of aerobics, kick boxing, roller blading, running, walking, shopping, or gardening don't work. Those exercises do burn calories, but only while actually exercising. Weight training burns and builds – it's a two for one special. By building more muscle you will burn more fat 24 hours a day.

In the previous example, Danielle's stomach will look much like it did before, no matter how much she uses her Gut Buster. Once she begins working her larger muscle groups through high-intensity, short-duration weight training, program, she will begin burning off the fat. Once the fat is off, those defined stomach muscles will be unveiled. In other words, in order to get fat off your gut, you must weight-train your entire body. Spot training (spot reducing) your abs will not get you the results you want!

3-2-1 Priority Training System

Busy people need to prioritize their time to efficiently get the best results. The **TNT System** utilizes this fact-based on a *3-2-1 Priority System*, to aid your training progress. This is the *fastest way* to produce fitness *results*.

Point values are assigned to body parts. The larger the body part, the higher the point value. *__Keep in mind__, that you burn more fat by training a three or a two than any of the ones.
3 Points: Legs, thighs, hamstrings, and glutes (and, as our daughter Jennifer would say; "your bumper")
2 Points: Back and chest
1 Point: Shoulders, triceps, biceps, calves, and finally, abs

In order to kick-start your fat-burning potential, *train the largest muscles first* in almost every training session. Also, don't waste another penny on a "Gut Buster" or any other piece of exercise equipment you see advertised on TV. Begin, today, by prioritizing your workout around the body parts that burn the most fat (i.e., legs, back, and chest).

Don't get me wrong, you still need to train abs. But, (and this is a big but) the only way for your abdominal muscles to become visible, is to burn off the fat, first by working your 3's and 2's.

If you weight train antagonistic (opposite) body parts for two 45 minutes sessions per week on non-consecutive days, you will begin to notice fat loss almost immediately.

Antagonistic (Opposite) Body Parts
Examples:
Thigh/Hamstring (3's)
Back/Chest (2's)
Triceps/Biceps (1's)

Afraid to step into a gym? Then your real issue is *fear*. Most modern health clubs have quality instructors available for any age or ability. Ask for their assistance. The issue isn't so much fear, as it is change.

Have faith! You are on your way to training like a pro and burning more fat than you ever thought possible.

Caution: If you happen to be more than 30-50 pounds overweight(nearing obesity), please consult your personal physician prior to beginning any exercise program. Reason being, most physicians will advise to drastically cut your calorie intake and begin a cardiovascular program before doing any type of high-intensity weight training.

Why? It is a more gradual approach to fat-loss, one which will ease you into making better nutritional choices and coax your body to change.

The Guts Needed to Develop Your Weaknesses

Arnold (Schwarzenegger, not Palmer) had poor calves when he first started weight training. His strategy: cut off the bottom of his sweat pants to expose his small, undeveloped (read: puny) calves to the constant ridicule of other bodybuilders in the gym.

The result: He trained his calves first in every scheduled calf workout and literally willed them to grow. At his best, his calves (now cows) were about 21 inches, and near the end of his Mr. Olympia reign, became one of his best body parts.

Hint: If Arnold could prioritize his weak points ... so can you! If you have a weak body part then train it first (most of the time).

Is anyone as confident as Arnold about improving a weakness? Yeah, right! He was the Terminator before we even had a name for it!

Targeting Weaknesses

The following chart will help you choose an exercise designed specifically to develop a particular body part.

Need	Exercise(s)
Shoulder width	Side laterals
Upper lats	Chins and pulldowns
Back thickness	Bent rows and machine rows
Lower lats	Low cable rows and one-arm rows
Upper chest	Incline bench presses and flyes
Lower chest	Decline bench presses and flyes
Inner chest	Cable crossovers and pec-deck flyes
Outer chest	Wide-grip chest presses and dips
Lower biceps	Preacher curls
Biceps peak	Concentration curls and one-arm cable curls
Upper forearms	Reverse curls and hammer curls
Outer thighs	Hack squats and leg presses with heels together and toes out.
Inner thighs	Leg adductions, wide-stance squats and leg presses
Upper thighs	Squats, leg presses and lunges
Lower thighs	Hack squats and leg extensions
Outer calves	Calf raises with toes together and heels out
Inner calves	Calf raises with heels together and toes out
Butt	Squats, Deadlifts, Reverse-lunges and stiff-legged deadlifts.

If unsure "how to" correctly perform each exercise, consult a personal trainer at your local health club or e-mail me at:
coachmike@drmbig.com

Chapter 6

Only, 90 Minutes Per Week ...
(Ideal for....Busy Baby Boomers)

Tales from the Gym:

Tom was a high-school football star, but you wouldn't know it by looking at him now. Tom is only 33 and he feels like he has the weight of the world on his shoulders. He would love to be in better shape, but he simply doesn't have time. He takes his gym bag to work every day and exercises at his company gym after work on the days that he gets off at a decent hour (which isn't very often).

Between a 60-hour-a-week job, three kids at home, a wife, and a commute, Tom barely has time to mow the lawn. His wife is a full-time Mom, so he has the pressure of being the only provider to his family. He would like to be proud of his appearance – or at least not be embarrassed to take off his shirt at the pool – but that's just not his top priority right now.

Fitness Solution:

Tom may feel like he has an excuse to be fat, but he doesn't. With 90 minutes of the right exercises per week, he can become a "Fit Dad." Tom's family and company would only gain by giving him up for an hour and a half a week. They will be beneficiaries of his increased fitness and self-confidence. Why do you think so many companies have on-site health and fitness facilities?

Weight training, first thing in the morning, will not only increase Tom's fat-burning ability, but also his energy level throughout the entire day.

It will take Tom only 90 minutes per week to go from flabby to fit.

Short and Sweet –
90 Minutes Per Week

A Highly Recommended Result-Producing Workout Regimen.

Day one: Squats. Try to use a "station" - the area in a free weight room where the barbell is attached to a sliding bar. Reason being, starting out, it's safer and I want you to be concerned with the feel of the exercise. Try for 2-3 sets to as close to "positive failure" as you can. After squats, try leg presses (2-3 sets) same deal. Use as much weight as you are comfortable with and take your time doing them (i.e. 2/4 sec. rep scheme – 2 seconds on the "positive portion" and 4 seconds on the negative).

After those two, you should be pretty well "fried," but if not try two sets of semi-stiff legged dumbbell hamstring deadlifts. That's it for day one. Rest for one or two days in between. Total time should only be 30 minutes or so after warming up for 5-10 minutes.

Day two (a few days later): Back and chest day! We are going to super-set (one set of back followed immediately by a chest exercise with little or no rest in between) everything we do today. Since your back is bigger... start with the back. Low pulley rows super-setted with dumbbell pullovers. Caution: Funny commentary ahead: a complete "puker" if done to failure ... but don't go that far unless you feel the need to vomit – just kidding.

After that, close-grip, palms-up pulldowns (seems like the same exercise, but it's not) followed by the station bar with incline barbell presses. Put the incline about 20-25% (not 30-45%... that's too steep an angle and doesn't work the chest as efficiently.) This group is a bit easier, try for 2-3 sets. Finally ... "breathing squats." Go to the free-weight bar this time, not the station. (We're working on balance, as well as control.) Reduce your weight (by at least 25percent) from a few days ago and try to go to rock-bottom squats with a lighter weight. Two sets only, to failure. Total time: 30 minutes again. You had better be breathing harder than ever when done, or it's not working right!

Day three (a few days later): Shoulders and arms. You will need that time to recuperate, rest and get this ... grow and get leaner. The reason you started this thing in the first place. Let nature work with you, not against you.

Shoulders ... one-arm presses while holding something up to keep your balance. Follow with tri-set fashion with press-downs (triceps) to failure, followed by hammer curls (biceps) to failure. Then, finally, rest.

Two or three total sets if you can. Do two sets of standing calf raises (12-20 reps to failure) and two sets of seated calf raises (12-20 reps to failure) and you're done.

Should only be 20-30 minutes here, too. Wait until you are around 15 percent body fat before you waste your much-needed time and energy on abdominal work. Why? Until then, you are working your abs every time you balance, crunch and hold your breath (especially on overhead presses and tricep press-downs).

That's it ... 90 minutes a week to be FIT ... not fat!

Piece of cake, right? Pun intended!

When in doubt ...
make the exercise harder.
How? Go slower or add weights.

Muscle growth is a metabolic response to an exercise stress given a sufficient amount of time to rest, recover, and grow.

Overload is a key ingredient to cause more stress. When thinking "overload" don't merely think of adding more weight (though that is the most obvious). You can also overload your muscles by:
1. Changing hand, foot, and grip positions.
2. Moving the weight s-l-o-w-e-r.

Suggestion: If you've reached a plateau, try changing your grip and moving the weight slower (allowing more time-under-tension, TUT). The added stress will yield better results!

TUT – By definition, time-under-tension (TUT) is the total amount of time the muscle is under stress – either positive (lifting), negative (extending) or static (holding).

Most workout programs (and a few uneducated trainers) don't spend a proper amount of time discussing/explaining this concept.

In most training situations, the body can hold 30 percent more weight than it can lift, and (better yet) can lower 60 percent more than it can lift.*

Example: You can curl a 100-lb. barbell ten times (to "positive failure") but can't do an 11th rep without help from a "spotter." If you could get help to lift it, you could still "hold" an added 30 lbs (for a total of 130 lbs) a few more times. This is called a "static hold."

Better Yet: Add another 30 lbs (160 lbs now) and you could probably still do the negative portion of an arm curl – lowering. Use this enormous weight until finally reaching a term (and pain) threshold, called "negative failure."

The Point: There are three distinct levels of "momentary muscular failure": Positive, static holds and negative failure. For the purpose of the TNT System, I will always refer to level 1 or positive failure as our goal.

* Dr. Arthur Jones , Nautilus Exercise Equipment Creator

Chapter 7

Nutrition

Tales from the Gym:

Amanda loves to eat. Among her favorite dinners are pasta and home-made pizza, with a spinach salad on the side. Dessert every night after dinner (assuming her veggies were consumed) was a way of life for Amanda during childhood. As an adult, she still craves that sugar fix every evening. She figures that she eats so many foods that are good for her – fruits, nuts, olive oil, eggs, spinach, broccoli, etc. – that she deserves a little treat every once in a while. After all, eating is one of life's great pleasures. Why should she be completely deprived of the good stuff? Right?

After years of on-again, off-again aerobicising, Amanda finally found a good gym with a trainer on hand to help her get started. Since she began using the 3,2,1 Priority System for three high-intensity, short-duration workouts per week, she has gone from a size 10 to a size 8. The only problem is that she wants to be a size 6 for summer. She doesn't want to give up her desserts – every time she tries, she just ends up binging.

Fitness Solution:

Amanda doesn't have to give up her sweets completely. The important thing about sweets and carbohydrates (carbs - pasta, bread, potatoes, rice, etc.) is that they be consumed early enough in the day so that they can be burned off before sleep slows the metabolism down.

Amanda needs to retrain herself to look forward to an occasional cookie or café mocha during her 2:00 coffee break at work instead of that slice of chocolate cheesecake after dinner.

The same is true with carbs. She can enjoy a good plate of pasta for lunch anytime she wants. That leaves the body plenty of time to burn it off. Of course, there will be days where dinner will be pizza or turkey with stuffing. The important thing is that Amanda worked out that day – which is the only way her body has a fighting chance of burning off the carbs before bed. **Her fat burning potential is at it's highest on the day of a workout.**

As for that after-dinner craving some of us experience, it's a matter of training your mind to accept a substitute - hot tea, fat-free frozen yogurt, raisins, a handful of peanuts, etc. Type and timing are key to eating the foods we love and having a body we appreciate!

Even if you're on the right track, you'll get run over if you just sit there.
- Will Rogers

Nutritional Secrets of the Fitness Pros

Long-Term Goal: Look good year-round.

Short-Term Goal: Be in the best possible shape on a specific date (a competition, a show, a class reunion, etc.).

Different food combinations work differently for different people. Don't say duh! You must get to know your body, how it reacts to certain foods, and what combination of proteins, carbohydrates, and fats work best for you.

For me this took years. Now at 39, I do very little cardiovascular exercise and still am pretty tight off-season (about 10 percent body fat) and carry about 235 pounds on a 6'5" frame.

• My year-round diet is a regularly 50 percent protein (about 250-300 grams per day), 30 percent carbs, and 20 percent fat. This is also known as a 50/30/20 diet.

• Water. Tons of it. Water, water everywhere! Most American's don't drink nearly enough water. You should consume a minimum of 8-10 glasses per day of pure water – more if you also drink caffeinated or alcoholic beverages.

With a higher than normal protein intake, you need more water to keep everything functioning optimally.

Contrary to popular belief, the more water you drink; the less you retain, and the more lean you will become and more fit you will look.

Have water with you everywhere. In the car/van, while walking, at the soccer games, everywhere.

Everybody is different.
Good nutrition is universal.

Supplements

Supplements work well when used properly, as a supplement to (never a replacement of) a nutritionally sound food plan.

Protein - I use MRP (Meal Replacement Powders). MetRx, EAS and V3S – there are many great ones to choose from at your local health food/nutritional store, or visit **www.drmbig.com** and order online.

- Glutamine – This is an essential amino acid to hard-training athletes. Amino acids (from 7th grade science class) are the "building blocks of protein." The largest amino acid in your body is almost entirely found in muscle. 60 percent of the muscle is glutamine.

- Fat-Burners - Ripped fuel, Ripped fuel extreme, Hydroxycut, etc. These are powerful thermodrens which raise body temperature to burn excess calories, so be careful. They are not recommended for anyone under 18.
  *And unless you do all the other things right (with TNT), *don't bother!*

- Protein. Try to eat some protein every 3-4 hours. How much? Depends on your body type, needs, etc. A range of 20-60 grams every 3-4 hours should suffice for most people. It keeps the body in positive nitrogen balance. That means it's metabolically active – building muscles and burning fat. I drink about half my protein (150 grams) each day, and eat the other half. Lean beef, chicken, turkey, and fish are good protein choices. Top vegetarian choices include soy, sushi, beans, dairy, and nuts.

*Most importantly, match your nutritional intake to your fitness goals.

Contrary to popular belief, the key to successful fat loss is not to starve yourself, but to eat something when you're hungry.

The best something choice: Protein!
Protein keeps the body's fat-burning fire white-hot!
If it's always burning, it's always working.

The Incredible, Edible Egg

Eggs are the Rodney Dangerfield of foods. They get no respect. If you want a high-quality protein, eat eggs. Think about it: You're eating a full complement of the essential amino acids. Eggs are also a rich source of thiamine, riboflavin, pantothenic acid, folic acid, Vitamin B12, biotin, Vitamin D, Vitamin E, and phosphorus. Seems like a complete food, right? Close. The only saturated fat is in the yolk (the "yellow" as Jennifer calls it).

Suggestion: For every 2-3 eggs you eat, only have 1 yolk.

Wondering where to get pure egg whites, without the hassle and time of separating white from yolk? Check out: **www.Eggology.com**

Another great source of egg protein is Optimum Nutrition 100 percent egg protein. I personally drink the chocolate version, and recommend it highly. As Dick Vitale would say, "It's awesome, baby!"

Go Nuts!

Most people shy away from eating large quantities of nuts because of the high fat content. Anyone who is interested in a healthy diet should not eliminate them, but rather enjoy a handful or two.

Most fat found in nuts is unsaturated (the good fat) – Macadamia nuts and cashews are two of the few exceptions. Nuts are also a good source of protein. Indulge yourself with dry-roasted peanuts for a snack and toasted almonds mixed in with your salads and green beans.

Fitness Tip:
Regarding snacks: Think substitution – not elimination. Nuts are great to keep on hand for a healthy and satisfying snack. I typically enjoy a handful after dinner when I crave something salty (peanuts) or sweet (raisins).

"Energy comes from the food you eat,
Motivation comes from the mind."

- Arnold Schwarzenegger

Fall In Love with Fish

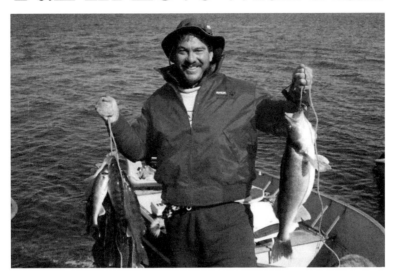

Fit Fact:

New research indicates that just one serving of fatty fish (such as salmon) per week can reduce the risk of cardiac arrest by as much as 70 percent. In a study done by the University of Washington in Seattle, researches found that individuals who ate the equivalent of 5.5 grams of omega-3 fatty acids per month had an associated 50 percent reduction in the risk of primary cardiac arrest. Four three-ounce servings of salmon contain approximately 5.96 grams of omega-3 fatty acids, enough to reap the cardiac benefits.

The omega-3 fatty acids found in fatty fish are believed to increase the levels of fatty acids in blood-cell membranes. This, in turn, reduces the clumping of blood platelets and coronary spasm. The study was featured in the Journal of the American Medical Association. Many tasty fish recipes are available at **www.Epicurious.com**. Check 'em out … just for the health of it!

Fish and Shellfish High In Omega-3 Fatty Acids (The "Good Fats")

Salmon (Atlantic, coho, sockeye, pink)
Herring
Atlantic Bluefish
Mackerel
Pacific Oyster
Squid
Sardine

Everything in Moderation

Well, Almost Everything

Nothing is bad if you don't overdo it, the latest medical research suggests, **except for trans fatty acids**, which are found in lots of cookies, desserts, and baked goods – and appear to be **really, really, bad for you**. If you're sick of hearing about what can harm you and **are ready for some good news**, here are some things that recent studies have found are **good for you:**

Alcohol in Moderation: An American Cancer Society study concluded that a drink a day cuts the risk of death by 20 percent (if you are of legal age to drink … duh!).

Socializing: People with strong social ties – those who are married, belong to social groups, volunteer a lot, have many friends – get fewer colds, a study in the Journal of the American Medical Association found.

Laughter: Two studies found that laughing has aerobic benefits similar to exercise. A Stanford University psychiatrist claimed that 100 yuks a day were roughly equivalent to spending 15 minutes pedaling a stationary bike and a lot more fun. Another study by a psychology professor at the University of Waterloo in Ontario claimed that college students' immune systems were stronger after they watched a silly skit. Laughter increases circulation, stimulates the heart and relieves pain.

Having a partner: People who buddy up with someone to reduce the risk of disease do much better than those who go it alone, a study in the Archives of Internal Medicine found. Couples who tried together to modify and control risk factors – cholesterol levels, weight, blood pressure, smoking habits, etc. – did four times better than couples where only one party made the effort.

Exercise: Pick your ailment – diabetes, high blood pressure, osteoporosis, depression, cardiovascular disease, stress, breast, colon, or prostate cancer – studies show that regular exercise reduces every risk.

> "Even if you consider yourself an intermediate, don't limit your choices of role models to intermediates."
> – *Mike Pierron*
> *Dream Big! Founder.*

The Most Important Meal Of The Day Is Not Necessarily Breakfast ...

It's the one that immediately follows your high-intensity, short duration weight-training session.

Why? Your window of nutritional opportunity is open for protein and carbohydrate consumption to aid muscle recovery and growth. In the long-term, this also means better fat burning potential.

The Best Source? Ironically, it's not food. It's liquid. Why? Your body is starving (literally) for good nutrition. Your window of nutritional opportunity is open for something easily absorbed (a protein shake) and quickly digested (i.e. liquids). A protein/carbohydrate mix is the best regardless of your fitness goals. Liquids make it easier for your body to absorb nutrition when your body needs it the most. Also, timing is critical for the cellular intake of protein, glucose, amino acids, and other nutrients. It's like a pit stop during the last lap of the Indianapolis 500. You need good, high-octane fuel for a strong finish. You are desperately out of gas – time for the best fuel available.

Motivation is like a fire, you need to continue to add fuel, or it goes out!

Good Stuff To Eat!

Anti-Aging Arsenal - A³

Food	Benefit	Substance
Tomatoes, watermelon	Protects prostate	Lycopene
Carrots, apricots	Neutralize free radicals*	Carotenoids
Potatoes, sweet potatoes	Boost testicular function	Protease inhibitors
Red meat	Improves energy	Creatine
Chicken, turkey	Aids testosterone levels	Taurine
Whole-grain products	Prevents Alzheimer's and heart disease	Folate
Peanuts	Supports sexual function	Arginine
Fish, olive oil	Lower cholesterol	Omega – 3's
Soy	Prevent cancer	Genistein, daidzein
Onions, broccoli,	Neutralize free radicals*	Flavanoids
Guiness beer – only 90 calories! Two a day if of age		Flavanoids

Chapter 8

Time to Get Fit

Time

A critical factor in achieving your fat loss goal is time.

Americans are so impatient. We try to do everything overnight. We don't see "fat management" as a **lifelong pursuit**. To enable the TNT system to work optimally, do not try to lose more than **two pounds** per week.

Since 3,500 calories equal one pound, I suggest you lower your calorie intake 500 per day (3,500 / 7 = 500) and add in 2-3 days of high-intensity weight training.

Result:
By simultaneously taking in fewer calories, as well as burning more, you are well on your way to an increased metabolism and enhanced fat burning.

To Sleep...
Or Not To Sleep

Arnold (Schwarzenegger, not Palmer again) used to call them "growth naps." He tried to squeeze in one or two small naps per day. Why? The body releases one-third of it's natural human growth hormone (HGH) when it sleeps.

Yohnnie Shambourger, 1995 natural Mr. Universe, realized the benefits of extra sleep the year his first child was born. His nightly rest ironically **increased** from five hours to seven and a half hours each night. To his surprise, this lifelong natural bodybuilder made astonishing muscular gains that year. (Hint: That's no coincidence, but rather more rest.)

"If you don't rest enough, you won't grow enough."

- Mike Mentzer
a HIT (High-intensity training) guru

I love **"weekend sports naps."** Turn sports on TV, and take a nap!

The benefits of sleep are many:
The body builds, repairs and replenishes itself during sleep.
Human Growth Hormone (HGH) is naturally released by your pituitary gland during Rapid Eye Movement (REM) sleep, one of four sleep stages that everyone goes through multiple times each night. The HGH promotes increased muscle growth and reduced fat storage.

Fact: **33 percent** of muscle growth occurs **while you sleep!**
You feel more rested, alert, creative and happy.
Naps are fun, free, and feel great – a true luxury (if you can fit them in).
Never sacrifice a good night's sleep for more time in the gym ... ever!
If you are not **fully-recovered** from a high-intensity training session, it's best to rest the next day.

Now, get fired up ... and go take a nap!

Chapter 9
Cool Stuff

An Interesting Body

I have an interesting body.
In a mall older folks sneak glances
when I'm not looking.
They work so hard to be respectful
and get their peeks in too,
But two-year-olds, they know how to look at me.
they linger as they go by, maybe even stop,
gazing at my three-wheeled wheelchair,
My bent feet and legs stacked like firewood.
They check out my hands and arms.
Eventually they get to my eyes.
Sometimes they have a parent tugging at them.
Only two-year-olds get to the eyes
that go with this interesting body.
When our eyes meet,
They gaze at me like God.

By Rich Foss
Plow Creek Fellowship

Planet Muscle

Jeff Everson, Ph.D., has lived an exciting sporting life.

Former editor-in-chief of "Muscle and Fitness" and trainer of six-time Ms. Olympia Cory Everson, Jeff is one of America's foremost authorities on advanced exercise, strength training and drug-free competition. His friendship and his writings have taught me well.

He also won the title I am working for, the Prestigious Masters (over 40) Mr. America.

Planet Muscle is his magazine. Pursuing muscle-building truth, this magazine is truly one of a kind – objective, honest and very funny. A rare find in the world of fitness and nutrition.

Training and nutritional truth are provided at a very low cost in Jeff Everson's Planet Muscle. It can be seen on Entertainment TV (E! TV). Check your local listings.

Call (800) 940-5978 for subscription information or visit them on the web at: **www.planetmuscle.com**

I wholeheartedly support and am also honored to write for Planet Muscle.

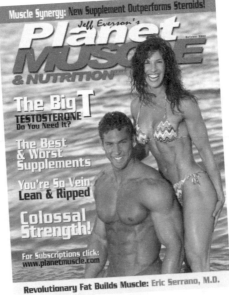

My Fitness Hero: Fred Grau

I met Fred back in the late 1980's and the first thing I noticed was how ripped and lean he looked. He looked incredible – better than most, if not all of the people at the local health club.

Fred is proud to be Christian, and reopened my heart to renew my faith. He truly believed that he could do anything.

He was a walking, talking, mountain of a man who impressed others (and me) just by his mere presence.

Fred was 53 years old.

Fred, now in his late sixties, lives in a suburb of Des Moines, Iowa. He continues to be an inspiration to fitness enthusiasts, and hasn't lost any of that great "newscaster hair" of his.

Here's to you, Fred! You'll always be the inspiration of my unending fitness journey. I can only hope to motivate others as much as you have motivated me!

> "Whatever age you can be,
> is the best for me!"
>
> *- Jennifer Pierron*
> *age six in a birthday card to her dad.*

Busy Baby Boomer – B³

After appearing on ESPN2 as Master of Ceremonies for the Fitness America Pageant and Superbody Natural Bodybuilding Championships in 2001, other offers began to come my way to M.C. fitness/figure and natural (drug-free) body building shows. What a fantastic opportunity to meet some everyday people who compete at an extremely high level athletically.

Melissa Stevens is one of these motivated women. She is a full-time mother of two from Elk River, Minnesota, and consistently wins or places in the top in every fitness/figure competition she enters. Her ...

Hobbies: Shopping, sleeping, exercise, and playing with her children.

Inspiration: To be a good role-model to her children as well as other 30-something mothers.

Nutrition: High protein (about a gram per pound of body weight – she weighs 125lbs), moderate carbohydrates, and low fat year-round.

Background: Cheerleader of six years and aerobics instructor for seven years.

She's fun, she's cool, and she's a fit mom.
www.Melissastevens.net

MICHAEL S. PIERRON

Personal Mission Statement

I am a husband.
I will work with, show respect for, and honor my wife, Linda.

I am a father.
I will be a positive person and a positive example.
I will encourage our children, give them self-confidence, and prepare
them to succeed in a rapidly-changing world.

I will seek business leadership positions.
I will continue to lead by example in sales, marketing, teaching,
coaching, writing, speaking, and consulting.

I will strive to build long-term, mutually-beneficial relationships
with our clients and suppliers, and to deal fairly and honestly with
everyone.

I will help our clients discover the best solutions
to their sales, marketing, and management needs by listening,
providing information, and performing services to the highest
standards of excellence.

I will live each day to the fullest
and adhere to the creed; the more people you positively impact, the
more meaningful your life will become.

I will laugh often and much
look for the best in others
and promise to leave the world a bit better than when I arrived.

Oprah!

I'd love to be your personal trainer.

Why?

1. You are "incredibly focused"
2. You possess great fitness potential.
3. You have a beautiful, natural frame.
4. Finally, and most importantly, the TNT System would work wonders for you. It was designed primarily with the busy executive in mind!

Chapter 10

Believe In Yourself —
Putting It All Together

Harsh Reality

The modern America is getting fatter and less fit by the day. Fast food, sugar, fat and chemicals are contributing to our fattening and lazy culture.

As a country, we are grossly overweight. We know better, but we ignore the problem. We deny. We procrastinate. We rationalize. We lie. We eat. We waste. We eat. We sleep. We eat. We mourn. We eat again.

Ironically, we find comfort in the overwhelming assurance of others, seemingly, just like us, who don't seem to care about our deteriorating health either. **The blind leading the blind** ... together everyone seems to be getting fat!

Stop the Insanity…
It Doesn't Need To Be This Way!

Getting leaner isn't a complex matter. While it usually takes time to find the interpretations that work for you, the essence of what you have to do is simple enough (read: TNT).

Being genetically typical and drug-free means that your most helpful sources of advice have absolutely nothing to do with the genetically blessed and the drug users.

- For competitive people only: if you lift Mickey Mouse weights, all you're going to get is a Mickey Mouse body.
- Focus on the big basic lifts and their variations: bent- or stiff-legged dead lifts, chins or pulldowns, flat-bench or low-incline presses, parallel bar dips, squats, deadlifts, etc. **Do this for most, if not all of your training time**. Keep your form strict and safe. Training right means not getting injured.
- Keep your ultimate goals big, and bite them off one at a time.
- Don't concern yourself with attaining outstanding definition and the finishing touches until you've built a solid foundation. Build the house before you begin to detail the porch (80 percent of your time should be in the result room not the cardio room!)
- Consider **abbreviated training as the first**, not the last resort. Don't waste years of your life trying anything and everything else before coming around to this point of view.

Key Points – Don't miss these!

- Get the body fat burning best by concentrating on leg and back work.

- Mistakes, lost time and bad judgments are part of the fitness experience. Learn from them and don't repeat them. Get smarter faster!

- Few people really train hard (i.e. with intensity).

- You never know how important good health is until you no longer have it. Avoid all harmful habits, activities, and environments (especially smoking!).

- Nutrition is about food, not supplements. Unless you have your diet in order and you're getting results in the gym, supplements aren't going to make a difference. Once you have a good working formula for training, food and rest, you can begin to think about which supplements to use.

- Taking supplements to slow degeneration and generally improve your health is another matter.

- Life is short and slips away quickly. Make the absolute most of it. Get in control, direct your own life, realize your own goals.

- It's not the equipment you've got that matters. It's what you do with it.

- Everything written in Fit Happens applies to women and youth as well.

- Never train if you don't feel rested from the previous workout. If in doubt, train less often.

- Different body parts need different recovery times. For example, you need more time to recover from a hard squat or a deadlift workout than from a shoulder workout.

- Abbreviated routines go as low as one exercise per workout. Three to five exercises are more common, although some hardgainers can gain from more exercises.

- Training a single exercise or body part three times a week is too much for most, if not all, fitness enthusiasts. Twice a week maximum or three times every two weeks is a better rule of thumb. Adjust it according to your recovery ability.

- A muscle isn't going to shrink if you wait more than 96 hours between workouts. For some exercises, at least for the hardgainer, the body needs more than 96 hours of rest for recovery and growth.

- If at all possible, have a like-minded (read: motivated) and serious training partner to push you each workout.

- What matters is what works. If you can only train on a routine that is by conventional standards absurd in its brevity and simplicity, fine.

- Never be afraid to experiment. Forget about what others think. Don't copy the masses in the gym that are getting nowhere and cardioing themselves to death five days per week.

Key Points – Don't miss these!

So often the less you train, the more you can gain -

...as long as you really pour in some effort and get plenty of rest and adequate nutrition. Try it. Just do the three "big" exercises (squats, or deadlifts, chinups, and bench presses) the next time you go to the gym. Do one to two warm-up sets and then two to four really hard sets for each exercise. See how much effort you can put in. When you leave the gym, you'll be tired and well-worked, but you'll have enough left to enable you to recover and grow.

Don't train through injuries. Always warm up sufficiently.

I can guide you to get leaner and stronger. I can motivate and inspire you. I can't, however, do your planning and training for you. You're totally on your own when you get to the gym. All the information will yield nothing unless you combine it with an abundance of diligence, planning, and determination.

Key Points – Don't miss these!

- Don't neglect your calves, grip or abdominals.

- Make progress slowly – don't rush it and hurt yourself.

- Cardiorespiratory fitness is important, too. Maintain at least a minimum of fifteen minutes of age-adjusted heart rate work twice a week.

- Want your training to work? Plan it to work, put in the work, and it will work.

- Patience and perseverance are a key element of achievement in anything, including fitness.

Partially excerpted from "Ironman" magazine, October 1991, Written by Stuart McRobert

Effort is everything! Anything less than 100 percent will diminish your chances for success.

Fast Fat Loss ...
Yeah Right!

Example: All of us have friends or relatives who have lost a significant amount of weight in a short time.

Questions To Ask:
1. Did they look good after the incredible weight loss?
2. Did they still have that reduced look one year later?

My guess is ... it's a gigantic **No!** to both. Why do they look like a "shadow" of their former self in a layer of loose skin? Because they lost the weight **too fast!** What's too fast? Any more than two pounds per week ... is **too fast!** They (your sickly, under-nourished friends) probably didn't weight train when they lost the weight. They, instead, got caught up in the "burning calories and not taking enough in" belief system and were **more concerned** with (and this is only a guess) **a lower number on the scale each morning.**

The Result: They were deprived of proper nutrition, and became fixated on seeing a lower number on the scale each morning. The dreaded rebound effect is almost certain to follow: Fit /fat, fat/fit, fit/fat, fat/fit...

The Point: Balance your TNT attack. Commit to much more weight training than cardio in order to raise your Resting Metabolic Rate (RMR). RMR is the rate your body burns calories at rest (i.e. sleeping, driving, working, coaching soccer, watching golf on TV, etc.)

*Weight training increases muscle mass helping to increase your RMR which **burns excess calories even at rest!**

*Hello, McFly!? Did you catch that?

*(National Strength & Conditioning Association, 2002)

Water, water, everywhere.

Fact: Water makes up 72 percent of your body. Drinking plenty of good-ole fashioned H2O makes you feel and look better.
(Georgia Tech Sports medicine and Performance Newsletter – Jan., 2002)

Sedentary people need eight glasses of water a day.

Others: (Read: hard training weekend warriors, young adults, baby boomers, teens, senior citizens and pretty much everyone else) need much more. How much more? A good rule of thumb is your body weight in pounds divided by two. For example, a 180-pound male needs 180/2 = 90 ounces of water per day - minimum. That's over 11 glasses!

Weight Training – How Young?
Most physicians discourage serious sports training in children because it could cause injury to the bone growth centers. However, weight training studies in children show that they can gain strength safely, provided the training is systematic and supervised.

University of Massachusetts researchers found that eight-year-old children gained strength better on a high rep program (12-15 reps) than on a low rep program (6-8 reps). The study suggests developing a "good base" is best for young children.

My recommendation: Ask this of grade-school children who show an interest in weight training: **"Show me how many push-ups you can do?"** Challenge them. Using only their body weight as resistance, (i.e., have them do push-ups. Wait until they can do 15-20 before moving to the next challenge … supervised and systematic weight training.

Heisman Trophy winner and star NFL running back, Hershel Walker claimed he never did any formal weight-training while in high school.

He merely did as many push-ups as he could every time there was a 3-4 minute break of commercials while watching TV each night.

I began weight-training to improve my performance in school sports at the age of 14 in my basement … just me and my boom box.

My first goal was to simply gain some muscle – I was sick of being skinny. I wanted to raise my self-esteem though I didn't consciously realize that at the time. I wanted to be somebody.

Confusion Abounds

In order to help you better analyze your thought patterns and make better choices, remember that every statement you hear is either a fact, theory, or opinion.

An absolute truth. Example: You burn 2-3 times more fat first thing in the morning on an empty stomach than at any other time of the day.

Working out every day is the best way to burn fat.

Swimming is superior to racquetball as a fat-burning exercise.

See how difficult it is to decide what to believe. It's actually confusing. Now, let's say an Olympic swimming hopeful with ripped abs and less than 10 percent body fat is the person who makes the swimming comment. He looks great, he's huffing and puffing and he just made an opinion seem like a fact, because it worked for him.

Multiply that by the fact that *you* have yet to find that "magic system" to help your fat loss efforts. You might become a swimmer on the spot based on a passing comment, (opinion), of someone who happens to be more fit than you!

Now, do you see how important separating fact/theory/opinions are? As the sayings go ...

"It's a tough job, but somebody has to do it!
If it's meant to be, it's up to me."

"My Grandmother started walking five miles a day when she was sixty. Today, she's ninety-five, and we don't know where the hell she is!"

- *Ellen DeGeneres, Actress*

Fit Happens at any Age

Age   **Activity Suggestion**

1-18   Team Sports, walking, biking, swimming, gardening, lawn care, car washing, shooting hoops, playing catch, and my teen favorite: kick-the-can – any activity involving movement.

18-64   Work and/or school, add high intensity, short duration, weight training 2-3 times per week (90 minutes total).

65+   Continue same exercise protocol.

Faith

Faith, the most powerful, but least understood motivation.

"With God ... all things are possible."
- Matthew, 19:26

Matthew didn't say some, most, almost all except fulfilling your fitness potential ... no. He said ... "With God, all things are possible."

Achieve
Your
Health
And
Fitness
Goals!

Fit Happens Success Formula:

1. Think it.
2. Write it.
3. Do it.

Congratulations! You're on your way!

Chapter 11
Setting Goals

You Are Not Alone!

According to many a Gallop Poll, the #1 New Year's resolution for 76 consecutive years has been to lose weight.

The obesity rate in the U.S. has doubled over the last 10 years.

The youth of today are growing fatter and have lower self-esteem than any generation before them.

Folks, we are going the wrong way!

Fit Happens... At Any Age was written in an effort to **reverse** the obesity trend in America.

The land of opportunity … is way too fat!

Goals ... If you want them to come true ...
Write them down!

What are your specific fitness goals? Think seriously about your goals and write them down. Make them big and challenging and attach a specific date to them.

Barriers to Success:
1. You
2. Your attitude
3. Continuously refer back to 1 and 2

Remember:

$$E + A = R$$

Education + Attitude = Results

Mind In Muscle!

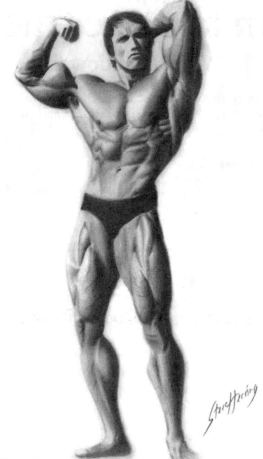

Arnold Schwarzenegger – arguably the greatest body builder of all-time– grew up in Austria as a skinny country boy, but trained his body and his mind to be Mr. Olympia by believing in himself.

Arnold believed (as I do) that the mind is your most powerful tool. If positively used, it can improve your fitness results dramatically.

Arnold was the creator of his destiny. He willed himself to be the best he could be. His powerful, winning attitude was one of envy. The command of his mind and his emotions helped make him the mega box-office action-movie star he is today. Check out his web sight: **www.schwarzenegger.com**

illustration by - Steve Herring
herring@maximumedge.com

Visualization

Visualization - The picture you form in your mind of exactly how you want your body to look is the key to achieving your fitness goals. Behavioral rehearsal is a form of visualization in which you picture the desired outcome before you take the appropriate action to reach the goal.

"What the mind can conceive and believe, it can achieve!"

- Arnold Schwarzenegger

A Better Way for Normal to Be

Feeling good and doing well can be a normal, rather than a "sometimes" kind of experience. In order to achieve such a way of life, "old stuff" needs to be addressed, and each new challenge analyzed and dealt with so that it doesn't repeat itself.

In a similar way, feeling good seems to many of us to be something that happens only sometimes. It CAN become normal. Aim for that, sincerely, as a new standard. Take care of whatever gets in the way. **Actively learn to feel good about yourself.**

If you are feeling incredibly wonderful, right now... how would your posture be? How would you be looking at things? How would you be thinking? How would you be responding to your environment? How pro-active would you be?

Remember... you can choose to be one of these ways right now. You can make this way of being standard, and start practicing making it "normal," now. Give yourself time, plenty of support and believe that final control (self-control) is within your power.

To achieve your goals, life may sound like a perfume counter – full of *Passion* and *Obsession*, leading to Joy!

How to Succeed with Clearly-Defined Written Goals

1. Be specific.
I will be at 5 percent body fat by January 1, 2003
I will compete in (and finally win) a natural physique competition.

2. A goal is a dream with a deadline! You must attach a specific time frame or someday will never come.

3. Forget realistic ... and DREAM BIG!
Don't ever place limits on your ability to achieve.
Don't ever set "realistic goals". (To me, realistic is another word for average.)

I'm not average, and neither are you!

"Most people are like wheelbarrows, only useful when pushed and very easily upset."

- Jack Herbert

Setting and Achieving Goals -
(pssst... The Secret)
Write Them Down!

Why?

Focus! Say to yourself, **"This is it. This I will do."**
It's **your** commitment to **yourself.**
It makes **you** accountable (again to yourself ... the person who you are trying to motivate)

Guess What?

The reason most people don't write their goals down is because **they do not want to be held accountable.**

This isn't a mystery novel.

I will not hide the answers.

I'll give you the fitness answer key.

Your challenge is to just do it!

"To succeed, jump as quickly at opportunities, as you do at conclusions."
- Benjamin Franklin

"When written in Chinese, the word "crisis" is composed of two characters – one represents danger, and the other opportunity."
- John F. Kennedy

The eight most important words in this book:

"Act as if it were impossible to fail."

- Dorothea Brande

9/11...
Where Were You?

The world changed forever on September 11th, 2001. Like every major event, none of us will ever forget where we were when the turmoil began and proceeded to unfold.

My own experience is even more surreal. I was one of about 50 people who witnessed the twin towers burning from the air. While on a Midwest Express Flight, direct from Milwaukee to La Guardia, we flew just south of the terrorist attack on Manhattan at 9:10 AM (Eastern Time) – approximately four minutes after the second tower was hit.

It was in one of those life-defining moments (and in the days and weeks that followed), that I made a promise to myself to live each day to the fullest and finally take control of this roller-coaster ride that is my weight!

Since then (at 284lbs) I'm now down to 228...
... and I can finally see my abs!

81 Out Of 235

What makes these numbers significant? I ranked 81st in my high school class of 235 students in 1981. That's 81st in '81 (By the way, Anna Kornikova's favorite number is 81 – not sure why I mention that, just thought it was cool, I guess).

Not even in the top one-third of my high school graduating class.

The point:
It doesn't matter where you start, it matters where you finish.

Fitness is the same way. It doesn't matter where you start, it matters where you finish. Have you achieved your fitness goals yet? Will you now? When will you begin? How about today?

Good, then write down your goals and begin!

"Impossible is a word found only
in the dictionary of fools."

- Napoleon Bonaparte

Chapter 12

Self-Esteem

Raising Your Self-Esteem

Tales from the Gym:

For 20 years, Teresa devoted her life to her family. As long as she can remember there has been a constant demand for her time and attention. Between working to put her husband, Bill, through medical school, raising two kids, and trying to be there for her own parents, the moments she's had to herself have been few and far between. She has always looked forward to reconnecting with her husband once the twins, Amy and Brad, were older. Three weeks after they left for college, Bill broke the news that he had found someone else. He wanted a divorce.

Teresa began to slip into a depression. Her therapist suggested that she begin exercising in order to elevate her mood and improve her health. It's true that Teresa's size 8 figure was but a dim memory. While everyone else was getting "Physical" with Olivia Newton-John in the eighties, she was breast feeding twins!

Teresa wasn't sure where to start so she began shopping gyms. She found one with a very helpful staff. A personal trainer helped her use the 3,2,1 priority system to plan her workouts. Before long, she not only had a nice physique but she also began feeling much better about herself. Her self-confidence skyrocketed, which positively affected all areas of her life. At the age of 42, her life is just beginning. It's time for her!

Why I Wrote This Book?
To Build Your Self-Esteem.

As an individual,
As a state,
As a country
And as a world.

*I believe how you feel about yourself is the #1 ingredient to becoming a
success in life!
Finally getting control of your fat loss efforts will give you more confidence
than you ever thought possible.*

You will feel invincible and it will "spill over" to other areas of your life.

You'll be ...
More confident
Happier
Have more meaningful relationships
Be a better spouse, parent, friend, neighbor, and classmate
You'll move closer to your faith
Your career will blossom
You'll volunteer more of your time
You'll have more "leisure time"
You'll reach out to help others because you have found the cure for your
fitness cancer

Congratulations on making the ultimate life-style choice for yourself.
The choice to live longer, happier, and healthier!

"Right now a moment of time is passing by ...
we must become that moment."
- *Cezanne, 19th century artist*

Huge flames mean huge fires. Light your bonfire of life today.

YOU CAN DO IT!

"The
   person
      who
         tried
           his best
             and failed…

  is superior
     to the
        person
          who
            never tried."

- Bud Wilkinson

Believe in Yourself

In their album, *The Grand Illusion*, the rock band **Styx** said it well:

You've got it all in the palm of your hand,
But your hand's wet with sweat and your head needs a rest,
But you're fooling yourself – you don't believe it.
You're killing yourself – you don't believe it.

Go ahead ... believe in yourself!

"The privilege of a lifetime
is being who you are."

- *Joseph Campbell*

Chapter 13
Attitude

Positive Attitude

You've got your work cut out for you!

According to the Zig Ziglar Foundation,
84 percent of all adult communication is *negative*.

And we wonder why there are so many bad attitudes out there ...
We're surrounded by negativity!

Positive Solution:
Visit our "Inspiring Greatness" web sight at **www.drmbig.com** and click on "GoalAchiever" – our all-positive, all-the-time newsletter. It's fun, it's a fast read and it's free!

Muscle and Mind Machines

There are over 600 muscles in the human body, made up of approximately 100 billion muscle fibers.

In fact, the body is more than half muscle. Muscles are used in every movement we make.

Muscle Machine/Mind Connection.

The human mind is incredible. It was estimated to be worth 85 billion dollars in the 1950/60s. – (Based on Earl Nightingale's positive belief system offered now at www.nightingale.com.)

With inflation…the human mind is now worth a good 250 billion dollars. Don't believe me? Ask Harvard dropout Bill Gates of what he thinks the mind is worth.

The secret of the mind … is making it work **for you … not against you.** Constantly giving yourself "positive self-talk"!

The statement, "Garbage in, garbage out" works the same with computers as it does with the mind. Guess what … if you "reverse it" and then **control the input**, garbage in, garbage out can be **replaced** with … "Good stuff in, good stuff out".

*Now, ready for the really cool stuff. *After 21 days of positive inputs, the mind cannot distinguish what is real and what was inputted.*

Highlight that statement and read it over and over and over … again.

After a while, the mind can't tell what was put there (intentionally by you) and what is real! Hello, McFly?

Does Visualization work?

Yes! Ask Michael Jordan, Tiger Woods, Picabo Street, Jennifer Capriati, Arnold (Schwarzenegger or Palmer) anyone who achieves anything really, really cool?

Ask them if they could *"see themselves achieving the goal many months and years before it actually happened?"*

I'll be willing to bet ... every single one could!

Guess what? It can, and will work for you too. But you've got to try!

> ## "You only live once, but if you work it right, once is enough."
> *- Joe Lewis*

> ## "If at first you don't succeed, you are running about average."
> *- M.H. Alderson*

> ## "It's what you learn after you know it all, that counts."
> *- John Wooden*

"A genius is a trained person
who does his homework."

- Thomas Edison

"Seeing tremendous growth
and positive change in yourself
can open new worlds for you."

- Arnold Schwarzenegger
Six-time Mr. Olympia

Chapter 14

Forever Natural

Steroids:
A Dangerous Epidemic
Just Say No!

I began my quest toward natural (drug-free) bodybuilding in 1987 on a bet from a friend who said:

"It's impossible for you to become a top bodybuilder. You're too tall."

To people who feel the same way and especially to today's youth: You **don't need drugs to succeed!**

Athletes, whether they are young or old, professional or amateur, will always be looking to gain an advantage over their opponents. The desire for an "edge" exists in all sports, at all levels of competition. Successful athletes rely on **practice** and **hard work** to increase their skill, speed, power, and ability. However, some athletes resort to drugs to improve their performance on the field or the court.

Some high school and even middle school students are using steroids to gain an edge, improve their skill level, or become more athletic. Steroid use is not limited to males. More and more females are putting themselves at risk by using these drugs. It's important to know that using anabolic steroids **is not only illegal**, but it also has **serious side effects**.

What are steroids?
You may have heard them called 'roids, juice, hype, or pump. Anabolic steroids are powerful drugs that many people take in high doses in an attempt to boost athletic performance. Anabolic means "building body tissue." Anabolic steroids help build muscle tissue and increase body mass by acting like the body's natural male hormone, testosterone.

Who uses steroids?
In the past, steroid use was limited to college, Olympic, and professional sports. Today, steroids are being used by athletes as well as non-athletes, in high schools and middle schools. Most major professional and amateur athletic organizations have banned steroids for use by their athletes. These organizations include the International Olympic Committee (IOC), National Collegiate Athletic Association (NCAA), and the National Football League (NFL).

Most commonly, steroid use can be found among the following groups:
Athletes involved in sports that rely on strength and size, like football, wrestling, or baseball.

Endurance Athletes, such as those involved in track-and-field and swimming. Athletes involved in weight training or bodybuilding.

Anyone interested in building and defining muscles.

How are steroids used?
Steroids can be either taken by mouth as a pill or injected with a needle. Of course, athletes who share needles to inject steroids also are at risk for serious infections including Hepatitis B and HIV, the AIDS virus. Some athletes take even higher doses, called "mega doses," in an attempt to produce faster results. Others gradually increase the amount they take over time, which is called "pyramiding." Taking different kinds of anabolic steroids, possible along with other drugs, is a particularly dangerous practice known as "stacking..

Will steroids make me a better athlete?
No! Steroids cannot improve an athlete's agility or skill level. Many factors help determine athletic ability, including genetics, body size, age, sex, diet, and how hard the athlete trains. It's clear that **the medical dangers of steroid use far outweigh the advantages of gains in strength or muscle mass.**

What are the side effects of steroids?
Steroids can cause serious health problems. Many changes take place inside the body and may not be noticed until it's too late. Some of the effects will go away when steroid use stops, but many do not. Male or female, if you choose to take steroids, you will be susceptible to the following:

High blood pressure and heart disease
Liver damage and cancers
Stroke and blood clots
Urinary and bowel problems, such as diarrhea
Headaches, aching joints, and muscle cramps
Nausea and vomiting
Sleep problems
Increased risk of ligament and tendon injuries
Severe acne, especially on the face and back
Baldness

Males:
One of the more disturbing effects of steroid use for males is that **the body begins to produce less of its own testosterone.** As a result, the testicles may begin to shrink. Following is a list of some other male-specific effects:
Reduced sperm count
Impotence
Increase in nipple and breast size (gynecomastia)
Enlarged prostate (gland that mixes fluid with sperm to form semen)

Females:
Since steroids act as a male hormone, females may experience the following side effects:
Reduced breast size
Increased facial and body hair
Deepened voice
Menstrual problems

Emotional effects:
Steroids also can have the following effects on the mind and behavior:
"Roid rage" – severe, aggressive behavior that may result in violence, such as fighting or destroying property
Severe mood swings
Hallucinations – seeing or hearing things that are not really there
Paranoia – extreme feelings of mistrust and fear
Anxiety and panic attacks
Depression and thoughts of suicide
An angry, hostile, or irritable mood

Above All:
Play safe, play fair: Success in sports takes talent, skill, and most of all, **practice and hard work.** Using steroids is a form of cheating and interferes with fair competition. More importantly, they are **dangerous to your health.** There are many healthy ways to increase your strength or improve your appearance. If you are serious about your sport and your health, keep the following tips in mind:
Train safely, without using drugs.
Eat a healthy diet.
Get plenty of rest.
Set high goals and be proud of yourself when you reach each new plateau.
Seek out training supervision, coaching, and advice from reliable professionals *(Step one: Read Fit Happens ... At Any Age!)*

If you, your friends, or any of your classmates or teammates are using steroids, get smart and get educated. Share this information with them and their parents. Take a stand against the use of steroids and other drugs. **Truly successful athletes combine their natural abilities with hard work to compete. There is no quick or easy way to become the best.**

For more information, contact the following organization:

National Institute on Drug Abuse *(NIDA)*
(888)-644-6432
www.nida.nih.gov/

This information was taken from an American Academy of Pediatrics publication.

Chapter 15
Attack the Hill

My Competitive Career
(If You Can Even Call It That)

1989 North American Natural Body Building Championship - Minneapolis, MN
Seventh place out of seven - (i.e. dead last)

1993 Prairie States Natural Classic - Decatur, IL
Sixth place... out of six contestants – (yep, dead last again)

1998 NPC Midwest Natural Classic - Madison, WI
Second place - out of two contestants – (dead last... again!)

I've competed every three to five years since 1989 and finished **dead last** for my weight class every time. Pictured below is the runner-up in the NPC Masters Natural Bodybuilding championship.

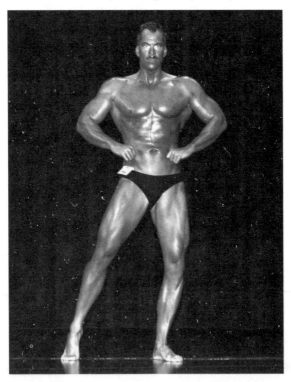

Question: Do you think I could have gotten into this kind of shape without a "positive competitive purpose" such as a specific deadline?

Answer: No!

Now, do you see why I suggest that you pick a specific date that has special meaning to you like...

An upcoming wedding
A class reunion
Graduation
An anniversary
A trip/vacation
And, heaven forbid, a natural physique, fitness, or a figure competition.

Ask anyone who has ever competed how they feel after their first contest. They will most likely tell you, "Fantastic – I looked fear in the face and did it, anyway!"

Kudos to all first-time competitors!

Less Than One Tenth of One Percent!

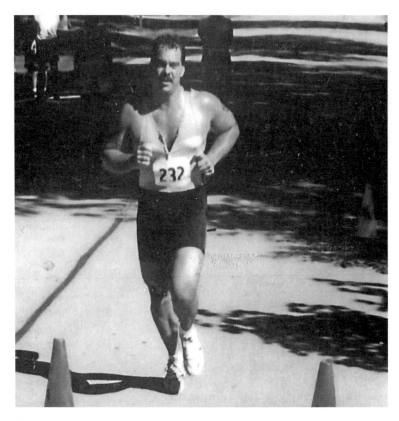

At the same time I began competing in physique competitions, I've also competed in four-triathlons! Once I broke through the fear factor, I felt that I could do anything!

> "Less than one tenth of one percent of the population even thinks about competing in a triathlon."
> *- Triathlete Magazine, 1992*

After reading that ... I had to compete!

Attack the Hill!
(My brother, Bob's bike racing strategy)

Attacking challenges in life is the sign of a winner. Arnold Schwarzenegger training his calves. People making presentations despite the fear of speaking in front of a group. Children trying new foods, making new friends, competing in sports, playing a musical instrument. My brother Bob winning triathlons.

His strategy is simple ...
Distance yourself from your competition at the toughest point in the race. Bob's "attack the hill" strategy is one of genius. Many less successful triathletes try to catch a breath when they are peddling up a hill. In contrast, my brother thinks, "I've got 'em now, attack when their down and put distance between me and anyone else 'gutsy' enough to try to hang."

"Attack the hill."

-Bob Pierron
Triathlon winner
1997 Sprint Series (19-34 age group)

The Result:
Race over! He demoralizes the field, and everyone else begins to position themselves for second place.

Question:
Do you attack the hill? Have you ever? Now's your chance...

Begin attacking your fitness hill now!

Make a plan, write it down and make it *happen*!

Godspell

My posing music at the masters Mr. Universe (once I turn 40) will be from the soundtrack of the original *Godspell* movie (1973 Arista Records - trivia: Paul Schaeffer of David Letterman fame is on the keyboards). My music is from the finale. It's a powerful, moving experience.

It marries the deeply spiritual journey you are about undertake in the physical feat of getting into the best shape of your life. During your journey, you'll laugh more, cry more, become more sensitive to other people's feelings and begin to change into the "new leaner and more fit you." The process will be life changing.

It will positively affect other aspects of your life (positive spill-over). Your career will blossom; you might get a promotion, a raise, or even offered a new job. Why?

You are **changing.** You are in control! Your attitude will get better, people will notice you, they may even ask, "What's happening to you? You seem different." Guess what? You are different!

Back to Godspell. It's time. It's your time. It's your time to change.

Oprah faithful, send her an e-mail **www.oprah.com** requesting a Godspell posing routine by the *Fit Happens* author.

"The mind, once stretched to a new idea, can never regain its original shape!"

- Albert Einstein

Chapter 16

For My Fellow Cheddarheads!

Fit/Cheddarhead Is Not An Oxymoron

Let's reverse the obesity trend in Wisconsin!
As of 2002, Wisconsin is somewhere near the back of the pack, (no pun intended), in state fitness rankings!

> *Let's reverse our declining trend and crack the top twenty by the opening day of the Olympic games in Athens, Greece by 2004.

My Favorite Oxymorons

Jumbo / Shrimp
Family / Vacation
Amish / Roadrage
Fit / Chedderhead

I'm very proud of my Wisconsin heritage. I'm **not proud** of our state's declining health and increasing sedentary lifestyle. We, as a state, are getting more obese by the day. Hey, we're fat ... with a capital "F"!

The irony: This runs contrary to our predominately hard – working German heritage.

Exercise In the Summer Months

In Wisconsin, we joke that we have four seasons: "almost winter, winter, still winter, and road construction."

Last year Wisconsin had a beautiful summer. It fell on a Tuesday.

The Point:

Turn off the TV and get outside for some warm-weather exercise. Lots of us are full of excuses: next week, next month, next summer, when I hit forty. It's unbelievable, it's also embarrassing. Fitness is a lifestyle choice. Make it a yearlong commitment, and begin today.

Stop it! There are no adequate excuses! None! Never have been, never will be. Get off the couch and into the game!

Your health and your kids' health depend on it! Your children imitate your every move. If you live a fit lifestyle, they will too!

Fit happens by choice ... not by chance.

One of my goals in writing *Fit Happens* was to provide the reader with a logical fitness system that can and will work for everyone.

I did 25 years of research and tested literally every training theory, did tons of cardio and almost starved myself into oblivion...then I finally figured out a program that I believe will work for everyone ... **TNT!**

In a way, you have hired me as your "personal trainer." And just like Tiger Woods (who wants to consistently improve his golf game with the help of his trainer, Butch Harmon), you have invested in me to improve your overall health, fitness and fat-loss efforts.

Now, as they say in Europe, "I'm going on holiday!"

Chapter 17
Value-added Fitness Knowledge

Elimination Day

November 13, 2001

To whom it may concern:

This letter is written on behalf of Michael Pierron.

Michael's last position was as a regional sales manager.

As part of our overall restructuring plan, Michael's position has been eliminated. This plan affected a significant number of employees, and the reduction is effective today.

     Sincerely,

     Vice President – Human Resources.

PS: Would you like to know how this feels? Substitute your name and the company you work for, where appropriate. Then as John Lennon once wrote …"Just Imagine."

P.PS: This actually happened on that exact day.

You're never too young to Dream Big!
(Fit Happens author, age 2)

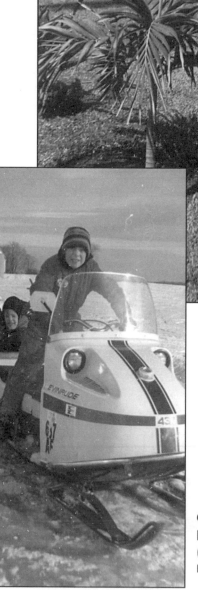

Check out that Evinrude snowmobile!
(Nine year old birthday party)

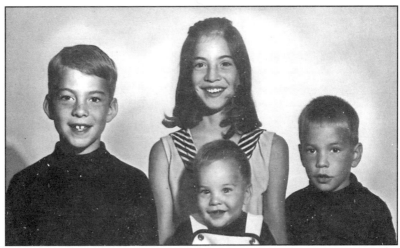

Church bulletin photo! The Greg Brady look-alike is me ... on the left, Michele, now with Sun Microsystems, Bob "the racer" at right, and Rick, the cute baby.

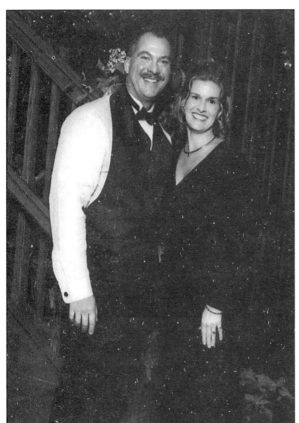

Mike and Linda Pierron at the Tinsel Ball.

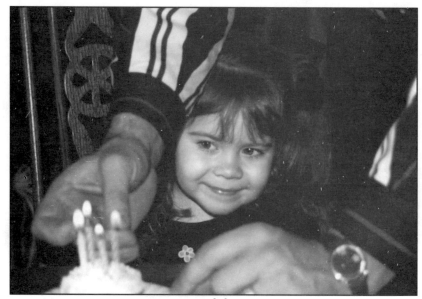

Happy Birthday Jen!

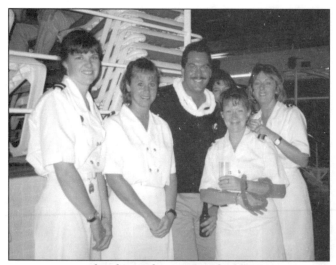

That better be a LIGHT beer?

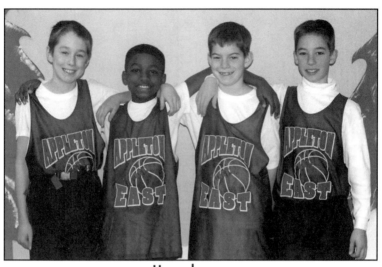

Hoop dreams
Johnny, Malcolm, Joey and Steven

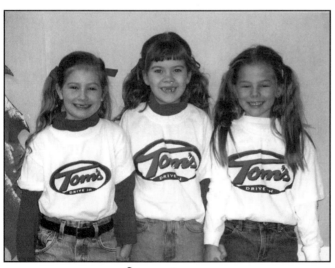

Soccer stars ...
Lynn, Jen and Anna

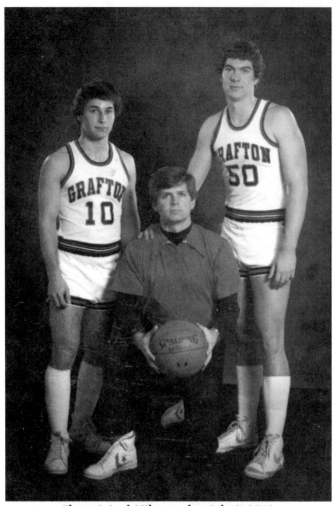

The original Mike on the right (1981)
6'5" - 195 lbs.

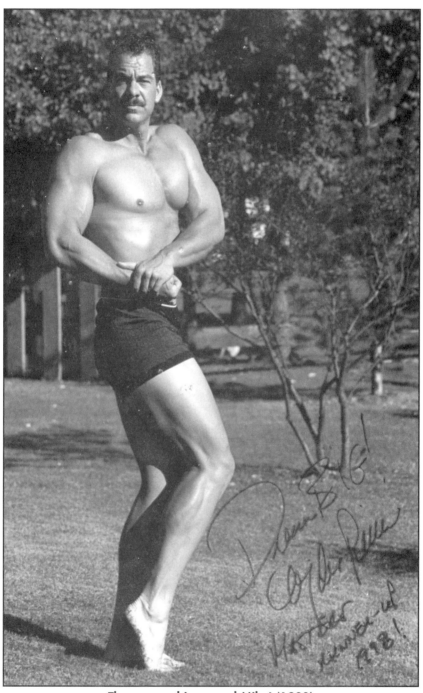

The new and improved Mike! (1998)
Natural Masters runner-up at 228 lbs.

Standing Ovations and Huge Thank Yous

To my wife, Linda, and our children, Joey and Jennifer – thank you for always standing by and believing in me. The best is yet to come.

To my parents, Francis and Barbara Pierron: Thank you for our family genetics, the ability to focus, the encouragement to dream and the desire to excel. I am very proud of both of you.

To my in-laws, Lee and Nancy Jones: Thank you for your support, encouragement, patience, and your daughter's unconditional love.

To my sister, Michele, for all the "snake-bites" growing up and to my brothers Bob and Rick. Bob who has raced everything from jet skis to motorcycles and Rick the funniest Pierron of the bunch.

To some of my former coaches: Bill Miller, Jim Miller, Mr. Ferguson, Mr. Meier, Coach Walsh, Coach Ohan, "Junie" Dickman, Larry Neve, Bill McGaw, Mr. Harms.

Thanks Especially ...
Dave Walker, Dennis Goecke, and Dave Dickman... for not only coaching baseball and basketball, but also preparing young athletes to excel in life after sports.

Thanks to our publisher, The Telegraph Herald in Dubuque, IA - especially Connie Gibbs, Marty Ploessl and Steve Herring- for his critical eye, creative insight and free-hand ARNOLD sketch"..

To Gretchen (and Robert) Forrester. At the eleventh hour she came through to decipher my handwriting, add creative input, proofread, and suggest critical improvements. This will be the first of many book projects in the next few years.

To Rick Berg, for a final professional proof (editor of *Marketplace Magazine*) before going to press.

Finally, to every person who said it would be "impossible" for me to compete in natural bodybuilding, because I'm too tall.
Thank you ... and enjoy!

Motivating the Motivator

Outgoing, strong-willed, gifted, and enthusiastic. These are words that come to mind when I think of my wife, Linda. Without her being who she is, I would have never developed into the person I am today.

Thank you for hanging in there with me ...

The best is yet to come!

I've Been Searching For So Long

-Chicago

As my life goes on
I believe somehow something's changed,
Something deep inside
A part of me.

There's a strange new light in my eyes,
Things I've never known,
Changing my life,
Changing me.

I've been searchin' so long
To find an answer.
Now I know my life has meaning.

Now I see myself as I am,
Feeling very free.
Live is ev'rything it's meant to be.
When my days have come to an end,
I will understand
What is left behind,
Part of me.

I've been searchin' so long
To find an answer.
Now I know my life has meaning, wow oh.

Searchin' for an answer,
To the question, oh yeah,
"Who am I?"
Maybe it's true, it's only nat'ral
Good things in life take a long time.

"I've Been Searchin' So Long" – Chicago
Grafton High School Graduation Song, 1981

Handout at a school assembly program

Success... Winning the Battle
Grafton High School - April, 1997

Throughout history, anything great which has ever been achieved was first realized in a dream. Once recognized and believed, this capacity to dream can have an enormously powerful and extremely positive effect on your life. We all possess this priceless ability, but it's up to you, and you alone, to develop and use it. Dream Big!

1.Visualization:

An effective success technique utilizing positive mental images and "burning" a subconscious thought into your conscious mind. A process in which you can actually "see" events before they occur.
Notable disciples of visualization: Abraham Lincoln, Arnold Schwarzenegger, Amelia Earhart, Brett Favre, John Glenn, Helen Keller, Michael Jordan, and Tiger Woods.

2. Your Sphere of Influence:

40 %   Parents/Upbringing
     *Develop a "winners" sphere of influence
 30 %   Experiences
     *Cultivate a never-ending hunger for new information
 30 %   The books you read/ the people you meet
————
100%

3. The Ten Commandments of Success™:

I.   Take Responsibility
II.   Raise the Bar
III.   Dream Big
IV.   Develop the Action Habit
V.   Visualize Your Success
VI.   Associate With Winners
VII.   Give Something Back
VIII. Embrace and be Flexible to Change
IX.   Learn to Love the Process
X.   Have Faith and be Patient

4. Motivation is like a fire, unless you continue to add fuel, it goes out.

5. The greatest advantage of having a "Goals Program" is the freedom of having direction in your life.

6. Most people, who fail in their dream, fail not from lack of ability, but from lack of commitment.

Four reasons most people do nothing:
A. Fear of failure - "Risk vs. Reward"
B. Poor self-image
C. Never fully understood the benefits of dreams
D. They don't know how to go about it

ACTION TO BE TAKEN:

7. Develop three short-term goals:

1.

2.

3.

and three huge dreams:

1.

2.

3.

8. Develop your "Dream List"

Your Personal Commitment:

I,_____, resolve to apply the Ten Commandments of Success for the next 21 days. Each day, in some way, I promise to move one step closer to my dream.

_____ _____
Your Signature   Date

Author Endorsements

"Mike has been an excellent art student. He plans out the total design first and then proceeds neatly. His use of color, texture, and line quality are excellent."

- Mr. Wood
Elementary School Art Teacher, 1972
Describing the author at age 9.

"Mike's projects show original thinking, organization, accuracy, and neatness. He adds much to our class discussions."

- Mr. Gall
Jr. High Science Teacher, 1975
Describing the author at age 12.

"The difference between the right word
and almost the right word,
Is the difference between lightning and
the lightning bug."

- Mark Twain

"The value of an idea lies in the using of it!"

-Thomas Edison

Inspiring Program Offerings

www.drmbig.com

Fitness/Nutrition

Fit Happens!
Motivating, inspiring and a once-in-a-lifetime type presentation. How does someone lose 51 pounds in almost two years? With a specific plan designed to do so.

How does someone keep that weight off for good? With a life-style commitment and constant feedback. You will never sell yourself short again, this presentation won't let you.

Learn both the "how to" and "want to" of improved health and fitness. (Hint: The answer has always been in the mirror.) Look and feel awesome and attend this program. The presenter is a four-time triathlete and runner-up at the NPC Masters (over 35) National Physique Competition.

The Future
What's New... in the Year 2010
Our crystal ball might not be perfect, but some trends are guaranteed to be with us forever. Discover the seven success truths that are universal and will be evident in every generation to follow. Learn them now, and share them with your family and friends and be permanently ahead of the game. (**Hint:** There is a reason that the best-prepared athletic team usually wins in competition.)

Be prepared to excel in the future... with this seminar.

Happiness is a Choice

Ideal for the "joy conference" of his life...this is Happiness 101 combined with Happiness 570. An excellent feel-good type program, in an era of the overworked, stressed-out, anxiety-ridden world we live in today.

Happiness is a choice. Take control over your ability to realize it.

Abraham Lincoln once said, "No one's happiness but my own is in my ability to achieve or destroy."

Make a choice today... and attend this session

Parenting

Raising Winners!

Mike and Linda Pierron present 101 proven ideas to raise "positive children in a world too often viewed negatively". Their book, Raising Winners, due for release in 2003, combines a positive upbringing with a current twist of dual career, information age, stress-packed living we engage in today.

The "Ten Commandments of Parental Success," are also unveiled in this encouraging, participatory program.

Motivation

The Ten Commandments of Success

This high-energy, motivational keynote is how it all began. A logical, systematic approach to achieving success in any endeavor is introduced. A fun, fast-moving, inspirational session designed to inspire your audience to "take control of their destiny." An ideal opening or closing session. Your presenter has the life experience equivalent to a "masters degree in motivation."

The Success Triangle

An ideal "quick start" to any program. Three of the trademarked Ten Commandments of SuccessTM are presented - take responsibility, dream big, and give something back. This 15 minute "quick start" sets the tone for your entire event. An ideal "opener". A proven commencement address home run.

Dream Big

Walt Disney was right... it all begins with a dream. A big dream. This session is a "grand slam, in the World Series of life". The best of the offering. Fun, fast-moving and inspirational. This program will permanently uplift your audience and prove everyone is capable of greatness. Caution: After this presentation, your group will forever be changed for the better. An ideal keynote address or meeting closer.

Change

Don't Think Change... Think Reinvent

Begin by forgetting "out-of-the-box" thinking and think "out-of-this-world". Ideal for companies who are under "massive reorganization". Constant change and innovation are the keys to long-term business success. This session will move you to recondition your mind and encourage you to bring your sledgehammer to work. Learn the seven secrets of becoming a "cheerleader of change". Caution: This program is not for the faint of heart.

Sales

Motivating Michelangelo

Motivating the super-achiever. Since it takes one to know one, this session is ideal for a high-impact, results-driven, assertive sales force who love risk. This program is designed to inspire both your top sales people and your top management to "think and act differently". Offering both the "how to" and the "want to" of continuous achievement, professional selling "basics" are quickly reviewed and a permanent "upward focus" established. Ideal for either the product or service industries.

Leadership

Leadership Secrets of Attila The Hun, Walt Disney, and Abraham Lincoln.

The essence of business growth is in the leadership of people, not in the management of them. Lead your team to new heights with less work on your part. An ideal program for new, middle, and upper management work teams. As all programs, "customized" to your specific goals and mission.

Teams/Teamwork

Some of My Best Coaches ...

Even though there is no "I" in team, there is a "ME". Your role as a team member, team leader and assistant coach - as it relates to both your career and in life. For best results: Combine this session with the leadership program and feature the teamwork program first.

You, Inc.

Is your "Net" Working?

Stay leaps ahead of the competition by playing your ace card today and everyday! Cultivate and develop your most promotable competitive edge, turn it into a powerful marketing message and deliver it to the right prospects. Ideal for entrepreneurial risk-takers. Discover the importance of the word "leverage." Learn how to increase the size of your address book.

Is this the end ...
or the beginning?

The original concept of this book developed out of an intense desire to inspire other people to achieve their fitness goals.

The motivational and inspirational aspect is huge. Equally important are the "how to's" of training and how that can be a catalyst to other successes in life.

> *Fit Happens* was written with **you** in mind!
> Only ***your*** success will determine the true measure of this book.

I sincerely hope that by first tackling fat loss, the most fundamental and universal truth, each of us will be held more accountable to our dreams and future accomplishments.

Remember… the most important opinion you have is the one that you have of yourself.

Dream big... and God bless!

"Fit Happens is a valuable program that will benefit anyone trying to better their physical, emotional and spiritual health."

- Jennifer Romagna
2-Time Boston Marathon Competitor

"Dad, this is really cool!"

- Joey Pierron (age 10)
Creative Director of Dream Big!

"Thank you for mentioning me.
I bet it will help other kids!"

- Jennifer Pierron (age 7)
Artistic Director of Dream Big!

"Keep pouring it on with Dream Big!"

- Harvey Mackay, best-selling Author

"Fit Happens is fun, fast-moving and
EFFECTIVE.
Just like a work-out with Mike."

- Cal, 48 and Kellie Watters, 42
Watters Plumbing,
Personal training clients

"Fit Happens (the CD)… 75 minutes of real experiences and real solutions!"

- Scott Mautz
B.S. in Exercise Science

"I loved it. I listened to Fit Happens on CD twice, then gave it to my wife to listen to. She thought it was awesome too."

- Mike Verstagen
All–Big Ten Offensive Tackle
for the 1994 Wisconsin Badgers

"What can I say… you inspire me!"

- Shelle Bernfeld
Fitness Competitor

"Mike Pierron is a cross between Tom Selleck and Lou Ferrigno… and he's NICE!"

- Susan Anderson

"45 minutes, twice a week, but INTENSE! That's how we work out. Mr. Pierron knows RESULTS."

- Paul Anderson, 17
6'6" senior
Appleton East high school

"YOU DON'T HAVE TO BE PERFECT
IN ORDER TO BE SUCCESSFUL."

–Anonymous

"Courage is a resistance to fear,
mastery of fear – not absence of fear."

-Mark Twain

"Being overweight and obese are among the most pressing new health challenges we face today."

-HHS Secretary Tommy G. Thompson

- Approximately 300,000 U.S. deaths a year currently are associated with obesity and being overweight

- In 1999, an estimated 61 percent of U.S. adults were overweight, along with 13 percent of children and adolescents.

- Change the **perception** of obesity so that **health** becomes the **chief concern**, not **personal appearance**.

- Ensure daily, quality physical education for all school grades. Currently, Only one state in the country – Illinois – requires physical education for Grades K-12, while only about one in four teenagers nationwide take part in some form of physical education.

- Limit the time spent watching television and in other sedentary activities.

Your call to action:

E-mail, phone, or write your local and national lawmakers and **demand physical education be restored in every K-12 school in the country.** Our nation's health is at stake – and our future!

Fitness results
This book will provide them.

Fit Happens … At Any Age is the first fitness book kind to provide both the "how to" with the "want to".
TNT System
3,2,1 Priority System
Ten Commandments of Fitness Success.

Take Responsibility: No matter how good your personal physician, the ultimate responsibility for your health is up to you. Apply the Power of TNT to reach your fitness goals. Learn proper Training, match your Nutrition with your goals, and allow Time for it all to work. Dream Big! Believe that getting in the best shape of your life is possible, regardless of your age. Develop the Action Habit and Move! Think priority management, effectiveness and efficiency. Invest in the Fitness Lifestyle. Understand exercise is a "two for one" special. For every one hour you exercise, it's proven, you gain an extra two hours of quality living. For best results…throw away your scale! It doesn't matter how much you weigh; it matters how much you look like you weigh. (Hint: Muscle weighs twice as much as fat)

Drink more water. Strive to drink eight to ten glasses of pure water each day. Become a Morning Person. You will burn two to three times more fat first thing in the morning on an empty stomach than any other time of the day! Think High-Intensity Training. Stick to basic, compound, exercises to burn the most fat, and add variety to each visit.

Motivation behind achievement of your goals
Sure-fire goal achievement system:
Think it • Write it • Do it

The author is a four-time triathlete and natural (drug-free) Mr. Universe contender. He's also the founder and Chief Creative Officer of Dream Big!, a performance improvement consulting firm offering creative motivational solutions to the universal challenges of:
Motivation
Change • Sales • Leadership • Fitness/Nutrition
You, Inc. • Parenting • Teams/Teamwork • The Future

Successful Coaching

Coaching is a critical element in today's economy. Our competitive environment has created pressure to do **more with less**. One of my goals in writing this book is to help you overcome obstacles in improving your fitness level, while teaching you to become your own personal trainer.

Dream Big! is a performance improvement consulting firm providing creative motivational solutions.

Also, check out: **www.thecoachingstaff.com** for additional life enhancing coaches. As a faculty member, I'm honored to be associated with such a fine organization.

About The Author

Michael S. Pierron is Founder and Chief Creative Officer of **Dream Big!**, a family – owned performance improvement consulting firm.

Dream Big! Provides creative motivational solutions to those who dare to DREAM BIG!
Areas of inspiration consist of

Motivation
Change
Sales
Leadership
Teams/Teamwork
Fitness/Nutrition
You, Inc.
Parenting
The Future

If you are looking for a creative motivational solution to one of life's universal challenges, you've found an enthusiastic team.

Jennifer Pierron – Artistic Director
Joey Pierron – Creative Director
Linda Pierron – Chief Financial Officer
Mike Pierron – Founder and Chief Creative Officer of

Dream Big!

www.drmbig.com

Change

Are you ready?

Are you willing?

Are you committed?

Do you have the guts?

"Progress is impossible without change."

- Joey's Dad

"None of us can change our yesterdays, but all of us can change our tomorrows."

- Colin Powell

"Constant change is the only reality."

- Sid Maluhed

America ...

The fattest nation on earth!

The land of opportunity has become the land of plenty (read fat)!

Too much of a good thing makes Jack a dough boy!

What's our problem?

We insist on "super-sizing" everything... duh!

More bad stuff = more fat.

Hey America...
quit thinking "better value" and start thinking "**too much fat**"!

Morning Exercise Rocks!
(For Best Fat-Burning Results)

Q. When is aerobic exercise most beneficial? I have heard varying opinions.

A. Cardio work is most beneficial when performed first thing in the morning on an empty stomach. The primary source of fuel for aerobic exercise is fat, but in order for fat to be used, glucose in the bloodstream must be low or depleted. When glucose levels are suppressed, the body will trigger multiple hormones that promote the breakdown of fat cells and expend them for energy. This becomes a multi-step process that can only be performed when insulin levels are low. My suggestion is to perform cardio first upon rising. If cardio cannot be performed early in the morning, I suggest keeping carbs absent from the meal or snack preceding your workout. This will allow your body to be in a low insulin/glucose state, and **therefore use fat for fuel rather than glycogen from carbohydrate food.**

Keep Failure In Perspective

You've failed many times before... just think.

Trying to walk, you fell.
Trying to ride a bike, you fell.
Trying to throw, it flopped.
Trying to catch, you dropped.
Trying to run fast, you jogged.
Trying to cartwheel, you couldn't.
Trying to drive, you froze.
Trying to speak, you blanked.
Trying to hit, you missed.
Trying to get fit, you got fat.
Trying to get fit again, and it happened!

Fit happens by choice...
Not by chance!

Failure ... (cont.)

Anyone who is moving ahead in life is always going to have setbacks. The only ones who don't are the people who have just given up. As long as you are alive and getting up and trying to do something with your life, you will have setbacks. Ultimately the difference between Winners and Losers and the key to long-term success is not talent or ability, chances or lucky breaks, *but it is the way you view and handle setbacks and adversity.* There are other things that might play a part, but the key to success will be how you handle setbacks, because sooner or later everyone has them. Losers see setbacks as the end of the road, while winners see setbacks as a bend in the road. This ultimately makes the difference between those who win and those who lose.

"Far better to dare mighty things, to win glorious triumphs, even though checkered by failure, than to take rank with poor spirits who neither enjoy much or suffer much, because they live in the gray twilight that knows not victory or defeat. The joy of living is his who has the heart to demand it."

- Theodore Roosevelt

The Process ... and the Results!

You will get leaner, harder, stronger and change shape if you train and eat correctly – but be patient.

Don't be satisfied though with average. No one dreams of being average. Set your sights on your utopia. The peak condition for your body type.

Be motivated by "the look" that you can create in your mind. It will provide the fuel (motivation) that you need when times are tough.

Keep striving to improve yourself. Life is not a dress rehearsal. You've got one chance... and you carry your scorecard with you for a lifetime.

Be proud of what you've done so far, but press on to greater achievements in the future.

Your potential is unlimited!!!!

None of us got where we are alone!

If you need help, reach out.

Reach out to a motivating individual who you like, trust, and respect.

Ask him or her how they:

> 1. Got in shape in the first place.
> 2. Stay in shape year round (if they do).

The TNT System has worked for me - a tall, ectomorph who got fat in his late twenties.

Properly applied, it will work for you, too!

A single can of soda contains 10 to 12 teaspoons of added sugars.

Nutritional experts say the amount of sugar in only two cans of soda can suppress the immune function for as many as five hours.

Result:

Sugar is cosmetically bad for you by increasing your fat potential – we all know that. It also can be detrimental to your overall health by compromising your body's immune system.

"Destiny is a choice.
It's not a thing to be waited for,
it's a thing to be created."

- *William Jennings Bryant*

Motivation vs. Frustration

Fit Happens contains 25 years of trial and error research in my pursuit of applying "logic and reason" to developing a training and nutritional system. To help America lose fat.

The Three D's of Fitness Success:

Desire – Your degree of "want to".

Dedication – Your ability to stick to a proven plan.

Discipline – Nutrition - your food consumption and supplementation strategy are a 24/7 job!

Keep Your GI Rating Down!

America's problem with obesity is directly related to over-consumption of severely processed carbohydrate foods and a wide-spread nutritional deficiency of essential fatty acids (EFAs). Fat-free refined carbohydrate foods are the deadliest kinds of carbs because they have a super high glycemic index. Simply put, the higher the glycemic index rating for a carbohydrate, the greater its potential to make you store body fat and ruin your health.

The following glycemic index rating depicts foods that cause a rapid rise in insulin, (the higher the number) which slows your fat burning potential.

Fitness tip:
Think "The later, the lower"
(Later in the day, try to eat the lower numbers on the chart)

Glycemic Index Rating of Foods

Food	Rating	
Maltodextrin (Worst Carb)	105	
Glucose	100	
White Bread	95	} Arnold called these two
Instant Rice	90	culprits "white death"
Pretzels (White)	85	
Rice Cakes	80	
French Fries	80	
Honey	75	
Sucrose (table sugar)	75	
Cheerios	75	
Ice Cream (low fat)	70	
White Rice	70	
Pasta (white)	65	
100% Whole Wheat Bread	65	
Banana	60	
Ice Cream (full fat)	60	
Brown Rice	55	
Sweet Potato	55	
Pita Bread (regular)	55	
Popcorn	55	
Oatmeal (slow cooking)	55	
Yams	50	
Grapes	45	
Pasta (whole grain)	45	
Green Beans	40	
Orange	40	
Apple	40	
Strawberries	30	
All lettuce (under)	30	
Lima beans (under)	30	
Skim Milk	30	
Fructose	20	
Nuts	15/30	
Yogurt (plain)	15	

Source: Anabolic Scientific Muscle Journal

• The lower the slower... *(its release of insulin into your system)* and the slower the better!

Have Faith and Be Patient

The tenth commandment of the "Ten Commandments of Success" is to have faith and be patient.

"With God, all things are possible!"
- Matthew 19:26

"We travel through life with a series of challenges brilliantly disguised as insurmountable opportunities."
- unknown

A powerful faith gives you both:

Hope
Strength
(and who couldn't use more of these?)

Patience is a virtue.

Our world is changing faster than any other time in history. Patience and your ability to be at ease with yourself in times of stress will continue to help determine how far you will go in life.

Most people trying to get fit…

…remind me of a person who tries "very hard" to get a suntan, but repeatedly makes the mistake of "lying out" at midnight. That person also tries every different supplement and training strategy imagined, only to become distinctly over-trained and in thousands of dollars in nutritional debt! - Exhausted, spent and confused - they quit!

The TNT System (of training, nutrition, and time) enables each person the flexibility to develop their own, best result-producing program wrapped around the fundamentals of:

1. Training with high-intensity, short-duration, and infrequent sessions using compound movements primarily consisting of, larger muscle groups:

1. Deadlifts
2. Squats
3. Leg Press
4. Rows
5. Pulldowns
6. Incline Presses
7. Lateral Raises
8. Push Downs
9. Dips
10. Calf Raises

These ten exercises have grown about 80% of the muscle known to mankind throughout the ages.

* Mastering these, on a high-intensity (near failure), short-duration (45 minutes or less) and infrequent (2-3 times a week) will do more for your fat-loss effort than anything you've ever tried before!

2. Nutrition is the toughest obstacle, but also the greatest change opportunity in attaining the look of your dreams.

*Food / Supplements

How much is a personal decision depending on your goals, budget, and lifestyle.

*Protein – To eat (and drink) protein is to throw a log on your body's metabolic fire. One log at a time keeps the body burning **White Hot!**

(Hint: That's a good thing for fat loss!)

Once you have sufficiently stimulated an adaptive response in the body via the application of a high-intensity training stress, adequate nutrition must be provided in order to "build and repair" tissue. That is the key to everything: building muscle, losing fat, becoming leaner, and looking and feeling better and being more fit!

Protein is paramount!

Protein, itself, is the only nutrient that builds and repairs muscle tissue! It is essential… Read: mandatory.

Think … "whey during the day!" Whey protein, like 100% whey by **www.optimumnutrition.com** is what I use.

3. Time. Rest and recuperation (the time between training sessions when nutrition has been consistent and with high-quality proteins) is when the body actually provides the growth (adaptive response) that the workout merely stimulated!

*99 percent of fitness fanatics have over-trained (myself included many times) in pursuit of the fit look they desire.

The real secret to making continual progress in fitness is to constantly monitor your body's feedback and recuperative ability.

"You don't rest enough,
you don't grow enough."

- Dr. Arthur Jones
Nautilus Equipment fame

Strength
(In review, to prove the point)

Between positives, "static holds" and negatives your greatest strength by far is the negative.

Most people who finally stumble their way into the weight room (I call it the result room) find most people merely lifting weights.

"Hey, are you goin' to lift today?"

What advanced trainers have learned, tried, applied, and now teach is that there are three levels of muscle stressing ability:

1. Positive or lifting, which is technically the weakest of the three.

2. Static or holding the weight, which is considered considerably greater than lifting or positive strength.

3. Negative strength is by far the greatest - about 30% more than that of even static strength.

Example:
A person who can Curl 100 pounds (positive strength) can usually Hold 130 pounds (static hold) and Lower 160 pounds under control (negative).

What does all this mean?
You can raise your intensity level by training first to positive failure, then do a muscle static hold – holding the contraction as long as possible. Finally, lower the weight under control to better stimulate and fatigue the muscle.

One pound of muscle = approximately 600 calories.

Muscle tissue is not mostly protein, but water – 72% to be precise.

Aerobic (meaning "with oxygen") has been overly emphasized in health clubs, gyms and the media because more people are willing to do aerobics other than "result-producing weight training".

Also, it's not that tough to walk, run, bike, step, stairmaster, row, etc. There is no specific training required. But, and this is a huge "fat bastard" but, as Austin Powers would say, **just because it's easier, doesn't make it better!**

Volume and Frequency

How much *(or how little)* and when?

To approach any type of advanced training (in almost any field or endeavor) one must push oneself.

Dr. Arthur Jones, the creator of nautilus exercise machines, has said of stress tolerance,

"Volume and frequency must be cautiously regulated because [human beings'] recovery ability is **strictly limited**."

Example:

Even if you are an Olympic marathon runner you couldn't possibly run 3 sub-2 hour marathons in one week. But that is what most people do by training over 2 hours a day at least three times a week.

In trying to speed the muscle-building processes and improve their fat-burning potential, most people grossly overtrain and generally under-nourish!

TNT Recommendations!

2 – 45 minute workouts twice a week
First thing in the morning for best fat burning results

Life-Enhancing Powers in Common Foods

Q: Every time I turn around, I hear someone buzzing about the Mediterranean Diet. What is it? The newest fad diet? Where can I get a copy?

A: The Mediterranean diet is not a new fad diet – there are no "copies" for sale. In fact, the Mediterranean diet has helped generations of people live longer and healthier lives. It is a delicious way of eating that promotes good health, rather than quick weight loss.

Research has uncovered that people in the countries bordering the Mediterranean Sea exhibit strikingly low rates of heart and other chronic diseases and have high adult life expectancy compared to Americans. This has prompted many health-conscious people to begin eating more of a Mediterranean-style diet, which includes whole grain breads and pasta (not after 4 p.m., please!), plenty of fruits and vegetables, fish, nuts, olive oil, garlic, wine in moderation, and small amounts of lean red meat. Also important to the Mediterranean diet is exercise and a high intake of something called antioxidants. An antioxidant is a substance that can prevent molecules in your body called "free radicals" from damaging vital tissue.

Food stimulates diverse biological activity. Here are the varied life-enhancing powers that have been attributed to common foods, according to the latest evidence. Not surprisingly, many of the below listed "power foods" are part of the Mediterranean diet.

Apple
Reduces cholesterol, contains anti-cancer agents. Has mild antibacterial, antiviral, anti-inflammatory, estrogenic activity. High in fiber, helps avoid constipation, suppresses appetite. Caution: Apple juice can cause diarrhea in children.

✔ Asparagus
A super source of glutathione, an antioxidant with strong anti-cancer activity.

Avocado
Benefits arteries. Lowers cholesterol, dilates blood vessels. Its main fat, monounsaturated oleic acid (also concentrated in olive oil), acts as an antioxidant to block artery-destroying toxicity of bad-type LDL cholesterol. One of the richest sources of glutathione, a powerful antioxidant, shown to block thirty different carcinogens and to block proliferation of the AIDS virus in test tube experiments. Also a vasodilator.

Banana
Soothes the stomach. Good for dyspepsia (upset stomach.) Strengthens the stomach lining against acid and ulcers. Has antibiotic activity.

Barley
Long known as a "heart medicine" in the Middle East. Reduces cholesterol. Has antiviral and anti-cancer activity. Contains potent antioxidants, including tocotrienols.

Beans (legumes, including navy, black, kidney, pinto beans and lentils) Potent medicine in lowering cholesterol. One-half cup of cooked beans daily reduces cholesterol an average 10 percent. Regulates blood sugar levels. An excellent food for diabetics. Linked to lower rates of certain cancers. Very high in fiber. A leading producer of intestinal gas in most people. (duh!)

Bell Pepper
Super-rich in antioxidant vitamin C. Therefore, a great food for fighting colds, asthma, bronchitis, respiratory infections, cataracts, macular degeneration, angina, atherosclerosis and cancer.

Blueberry
Acts as an unusual type of antibiotic by blocking attachment of bacteria that cause urinary tract infections. Contains chemicals that curb diarrhea. Also antiviral activity and high in natural aspirin.

✔ Broccoli
A spectacular and unique package of versatile disease-fighters. Abundant in numerous strong, well-known antioxidants. Extremely high in anti-cancer activity, particularly against lung, colon, and breast cancers. It speeds up removal of estrogen from the body, helping suppress breast cancer. Rich in cholesterol-reducing fiber. Has antiviral, anti-ulcer activity. A super source of chromium that helps regulate insulin and blood sugar. Note: cooking and processing destroys some of the benefit, it's best eaten raw or lightly cooked (as in stir-frying and microwaving).

Brussels Sprouts

As one of the cruciferous family, possesses some of the same powers as broccoli and cabbage. Definitely anti-cancer, estrogenic and packed with various antioxidants and indoles.

Cabbage

Revered in ancient Rome as a cancer cure. Contains numerous anti-cancer and antioxidant compounds. Speeds up estrogen metabolism, is thought to help block breast cancer and suppress growth of polyps, a prelude to colon cancer. In studies, eating cabbage more than once a week cut men's colon cancer odds 66 percent. As little as two daily tablespoons of cooked cabbage protected against stomach cancer. Contains anti-ulcer compounds; cabbage juice helps heal ulcers in humans. Has antibacterial and anti-viral powers. Like broccoli, the benefit decreases the more it is cooked. Raw cabbage, as in cole slaw, appears to have stronger overall pharmacological activity.

✔ Carrots

A super food source of beta carotene, a powerful anti-cancer, artery-protecting, immune-boosting, infection-fighting antioxidant with wide protective powers. A carrot a day slashed stroke rates in women by 68 percent. One medium carrot's worth of beta carotene cuts lung cancer risk in half, even among formerly heavy smokers. High doses of beta carotene, as found in carrots, substantially reduces odds of degenerative eye diseases-cataracts and macular degeneration-as well as chest pain (angina). Carrots' high soluble fiber depresses blood cholesterol, promotes regularity. Note: Cooking does not destroy beta carotene; in fact, light cooking can make it easier for the body to absorb.

Cauliflower

A member of the famous cruciferous family, it contains many of the same cancer-fighting, hormone-regulating compounds as its cousins, broccoli and cabbage. Specifically thought to help ward off breast and colon cancers. Note: Heavy cooking destroys some pharmacological activity.

Celery

A traditional Vietnamese remedy for high blood pressure. Celery compounds reduce blood pressure in animals. Comparable human dose: two to four stalks a day. Also has a mild diuretic effect. Contains eight different families of anti-cancer compounds. Eating celery before or after vigorous exercise can induce mild to serious allergic reactions in some.

Chili Peppers

Revs up the blood-clot-dissolving system, opens up sinuses and air passages, breaks up mucus in the lungs, acts as an expectorant or decongestant, helps prevent bronchitis, emphysema and stomach ulcers. Most of chili pepper's pharmacological activity is credited to capsaicin (from the Latin "to bite"), the compound that makes the pepper taste hot. Capsaicin is also a potent painkiller, alleviating headaches when inhaled, and joint pain when injected. Hot paprika made from peppers is high in natural aspirin. Antibacterial, antioxidant activity. Putting hot chili sauce on food also speeds up metabolism, burning off calories. Chili peppers do not harm the stomach lining or promote ulcers.

✔ Chocolate

Contains chemicals thought to affect neurotransmitters in the brain. Added to milk, chocolate helps counteract lactose intolerance. Chocolate does not seem to raise cholesterol or cause or aggravate acne. Dark chocolate is very high in copper, which may help ward off cardiovascular disease. Triggers headaches in some. Aggravates heartburn. Implicated in cystic breast disease.

Cinnamon

A strong stimulator of insulin activity, plus potentially helpful for those with Type II diabetes. Mild anticoagulant activity.

Cloves

Long used to kill the pain of toothache and as an anti-inflammatory against rheumatic diseases.

Coffee

Most, but not all, of coffee's pharmacological impact comes from its high concentration of caffeine, a psychoactive drug of great power. Caffeine, depending on the individual, can be a mood elevator and a mental energizer. One cup of morning coffee gives the brain a "jump start." Caffeine is an emergency remedy for asthma. Also, regular coffee drinkers have less asthma and wheezing. Dilates bronchial passages. Mildly addictive. Triggers headaches, anxiety and panic attacks in some. In excess may cause psychiatric disturbances. Definitely promotes insomnia. Coffee stimulates stomach acid secretion (both caffeinated and decaf). Can aggravate heartburn.

No solid evidence links coffee or caffeine to cancers. Caffeine may promote fibrocystic breast disease in some women. There's scant evidence of cardiovascular danger from moderate caffeine and coffee – under four to six cups per day. Coffee brewed by the drip method appears to have little or no detrimental impact on blood cholesterol.

WHERE YOU GET CAFFEINE

Food or Beverage   **Avg. Milligrams**

Coffee – 5 fluid ounces (a small cup)
   Brewed
      Drip   115
      Percolated   80
      Decaffeinated   3
   Instant
      Regular   65
      Decaffeinated   2

Tea – 5 fluid ounces
   Steeped
      U.S. brands   40
      Imported brands   60
   Instant – 1 tsp. instant powder   30

Soft Drinks
   Cola (regular and diet)   46
   Mountain Dew   54

Chocolate
   Cocoa beverage – 5-ounce cup   4
   Milk chocolate – 1 cup   6
   Dark chocolate, semisweet-1 ounce   20

Collard Greens
Full of diverse anticancer, antioxidant compounds, including lutein, vitamin C, beta carotene. In animals blocks the spread of breast cancer. Like other leafy green vegetables, associated with low rates of all cancers. High in oxalates, not recommended for those with kidney stones.

✔ Corn
Anticancer and antiviral activity, possibly induced by corn's content of protease inhibitors. Has estrogen-boosting capabilities. A very common cause of food intolerance linked to symptoms of rheumatoid arthritis, irritable bowel syndrome, headaches and migraine-related epilepsy in children.

Cranberries
Strong antibiotic properties with unusual abilities to prevent infectious bacteria from sticking to cells lining the bladder and urinary tract. Thus, it helps prevent recurring urinary tract (bladder) infections. Also has antiviral activity.

Dates
High in natural aspirin. Has laxative effect. Dried fruits, including dates, are linked to lower rates of certain cancers, especially pancreatic cancer. Contains compounds that may cause headaches in susceptible individuals.

Eggplant
Eggplant substances made into a topical cream medication have been used to treat skin cancers such as basal cell carcinoma, according to Australian researchers. Also, eating eggplant may lower blood cholesterol and help counteract some detrimental effects of fatty foods. Eggplant is also antibacterial and diuretic.

Figs
Long used in folklore to fight cancer. Has helped shrink tumors in humans, according to Japanese tests. Also laxative, anti-ulcer, antibacterial and antiparasitic. Triggers headaches in some people.

✔ Fish and Fish Oil
An exceedingly remarkable therapeutic and preventive food. Intervenes in heart disease, preventing heart attack deaths (two servings per week); an ounce a day has been shown to cut risk of heart attacks 50 percent. Oil in fish can relieve symptoms of rheumatoid arthritis, osteoarthritis, asthma, psoriasis, high blood pressure, Raynaud's disease, migraine headaches, ulcerative colitis, and possibly multiple scle-

rosis. May help ward off strokes. A known anti-inflammatory agent and anticoagulant. Raises good type HDL cholesterol. Slashes triglycerides dramatically. May help guard against development of glucose intolerance and Type II diabetes. Some fish are high in antioxidants, such as selenium and co-enzyme Q-10. Exhibits anticancer activity especially in blocking development of colon cancer and spread of breast cancer. Best choices include sardines, mackerel, herring, salmon, and tuna.

✔ Garlic

An all-around wonder drug, used to treat an array of ills since the dawn of civilization. Combats bacteria, intestinal parasites and viruses. In high doses it has cured encephalitis. Lowers blood pressure and cholesterol, discourages dangerous blood clotting. Two or three cloves a day cut the odds of subsequent heart attacks in half in heart patients. Tops the National Cancer Institute's list as a potential cancer-preventive food – especially for preventing stomach cancer. A good cold medication. Boost immune responses. Helps relieve gas, has antidiarrheal, estrogenic and diuretic activity. Appears to lift mood and has a mild calming effect. Eat garlic both raw and cooked for all-around health insurance.

Ginger

Used for centuries in Asia to treat nausea, vomiting, headache, chest congestion, cholera, colds, diarrhea, stomach ache, rheumatism, and nervous diseases. Ginger is a proven anti-nausea, anti-motion sickness remedy that matches or surpasses drugs such as Dramamine. Helps thwart and prevent migraine headaches and osteoarthritis. Relieves symptoms of rheumatoid arthritis. Acts as an antithrombotic and anti-inflammatory agent in humans; is an antibiotic in test tubes (kills salmonella and staph bacteria), and an anti-ulcer agent in animals. Also, has anti-depressant, antidiarrheal and strong antioxidant activity. Ranks very high in anticancer activity.

✔ Grapes

A rich storehouse of antioxidant, anticancer compounds. Red grapes are high in antioxidant quercetin and are antibacterial and antiviral in test tubes.

Grapefruit

The pulp contains a unique pectin (in membrane and juice sacs – not in juice) that lowers blood cholesterol and reverses atherosclerosis (clogged arteries) in animals. Has anticancer activity and appears particularly protective against stomach and pancreatic cancer. The juice is antiviral. High in various antioxidants, especially disease-fighting vitamin C. May aggravate heartburn.

Honey
Strong antibiotic properties. Has sleep-inducing sedative and tranquilizing properties. Never feed honey to a baby; there is a danger of potentially deadly botulism.

Kiwi Fruit
Commonly prescribed in Chinese traditional medicine to treat stomach and breast cancer. High in vitamin C, which has multiple antidisease activity.

Melons (green and yellow, such as cantaloupe and honeydew)
Anticoagulant (blood-thinning) activity. Orange melons contain antioxidant beta carotene.

✔ Milk
Cancer-fighting powers, possibly against colon, lung, stomach and cervical cancers, especially in low-fat milk. One study detected less cancer among low-fat milk drinkers than non-fat milk drinkers. May help prevent high blood pressure. Skim milk may lower blood cholesterol. Milk fat promotes cancer and heart disease.

Mushrooms (Asian, including shiitake)
Long esteemed in Asia as a longevity tonic, heart medicine and cancer remedy. Current tests show Asian mushrooms, such as shiitake, help prevent and/or treat cancer, viral diseases, such as influenza and polio, high blood cholesterol, sticky blood platelets and high blood pressure. Eaten daily can cut cholesterol. Contains a broad-spectrum antiviral agent that boosts immune function. Used to treat leukemia in China and breast cancer in Japan. Shiitake extract has been declared by Japanese scientist more effective as an AIDS drug than AZT. Eating black mo-er ("tree ear") mushroom "thins the blood." Note; No benefits are known for the common U.S. button mushroom, and some claim it has cancer-causing potential unless cooked. This somewhat contradicts the info in the below table that lists mushrooms as one of the 100 top bodybuilding foods. GCF

Mustard (including horseradish)
Recognized for centuries as a decongestant and expectorant. Helps break up mucus in air passages. A good remedy for congestion caused by colds and sinus problems. Also antibacterial. Revs up metabolism, burning off extra calories.

✔ Nuts
Anticancer and heart-protective properties. A key food among Seventh-Day Adventists, known for their low rates of heart disease. Walnuts and

almonds help reduce cholesterol and protect arteries from damage. Nuts are generally high in antioxidant vitamin E, shown to protect against chest pain and artery damage. Brazil nuts are rich in selenium, an antioxidant linked to lower rates of heart disease and cancer. Walnuts contain an antioxidant, cancer fighter, and are high in "good fat". Nuts have been found lacking in the diets of those who later develop Parkinson's disease. Peanuts are a prime cause of allergic reactions in some.

Oats
Helps stabilize blood sugar and is estrogenic and antioxidant. Can lower cholesterol in some. Oats may also help combat nicotine cravings and have antidepressant powers. High doses can cause gas in some.

✔ Olive oil
An artery protector that lowers "bad" cholesterol without lowering "good" cholesterol. Protects arteries from plaque. Reduces blood pressure, helps regulate blood sugar. Has potent antioxidant activity. May help ward off cancer.

✔ Onions (including chives, shallots, scallions, leeks)
One of civilizations oldest medicines, reputed to cure virtually everything. An exceptionally strong antioxidant. Full of numerous anticancer agents, blocks cancer dramatically in animals. Specifically linked to inhibiting human stomach cancer. Thins the blood, lowers cholesterol, raises "good" cholesterol, wards off blood clots, fights asthma, chronic bronchitis, hay fever, diabetes, atherosclerosis and infections. Anti-inflammatory, antibiotic, and antiviral.

Oranges
A complete package of every class of natural cancer-inhibitor known – carotenoids, terpenes and flavonoids. Also rich in antioxidant vitamin C and beta carotene. Specifically tied to lower rates of pancreatic cancer and may help ward off asthma attacks, bronchitis, breast cancer, stomach cancer, atherosclerosis, gum disease, and boost fertility.

Parsley
Anticancer because of its high concentrations of antioxidants. Can help detoxify and neutralize certain carcinogens. Has diuretic activity.

✔ Pineapples
Suppresses inflammation, aids digestion, helps dissolve blood clots prevents osteoporosis and bone fractures. It is also antibacterial and antiviral and mildly estrogenic.

Plums
Antibacterial, antiviral, and works as a laxative.

✔ Potato (white)
Contains anticancer protease inhibitors. May help prevent high blood pressure and strokes. Some estrogenic activity.

Prunes
A well-known laxative. High in fiber, sorbitol and natural aspirin.

Pumpkin
Extremely high in beta carotene, the antioxidant reputed to help ward off numerous health problems, including heart attacks, cancer, and cataracts.

Raspberries
Has antiviral, anticancer activity. High in natural aspirin.

✔ Rice
Antidiarrheal, anticancer activity. Like other seeds, contains anticancer protease inhibitors. Rice bran is excellent against constipation, lowers cholesterol and tends to block development of kidney stones.

Rhubarb
Extremely high in oxalates which help promote formation of kidney stones in susceptible individuals. Little or no laxative effect.

Seaweed and Kelp (brown or Laminaria type seaweed)
Antibacterial and antiviral activity in brown Laminaria type seaweed known as kelp. It kills herpes virus, for example. Kelp may also lower blood pressure and cholesterol. Wakame boosts immune functioning. Nori kills bacterial and seems to help heal ulcers. A chemical from wakame seaweed is a clot-buster, in one test twice as powerful as the common drug heparin. Most types of seaweed have anticancer activity. Seaweed is very high in iodine and might aggravate acne flare-ups.

Soybeans
Packed with pharmacological activity. Rich in hormones, it boosts estrogen levels in postmenopausal women. Believed to have anticancer activity – especially breast and prostate cancers. Soybeans are the richest source of potent protease inhibitors which are anticancer, antiviral agents. In many human tests, soybeans lower blood cholesterol. In animals, soybeans seem to deter and help dissolve kidney stones.

172 ───────────── **Fit Happens** ... *At Any Age*
✔ **Spinach**

Tops the list, along with other green leafy vegetables, as a food most eaten by people who don't get cancer. A super source of antioxidants and cancer antagonists, containing more than four times more beta carotene and three times more lutein than broccoli, for example. Rich in fiber that helps lower blood cholesterol. Extremely high in oxalate, thus, not recommended for people with kidney stones. Note: Some of its antioxidants are destroyed by cooking. Eat raw or lightly cooked. Prefer iceberg lettuce salads? Develop a taste for spinach by mixing the two and gradually increasing the proportion of spinach. Once you develop a taste for spinach salads, you'll never buy the nutritionally-void iceberg lettuce again.

Strawberries

Antiviral, anticancer activity. Often eaten by people less likely to develop all types of cancer.

✔ **Sweet Potato** (yams)

A blockbuster source of the antioxidant beta carotene, linked to preventing heart disease, cataracts, strokes and numerous cancers.

Tea (including black, oolong and green tea, not herbal teas)

Amazing and diverse pharmacological activity, mainly due to catechins. Tea acts as an anticoagulant, artery protector, antibiotic, anti-ulcer agent, cavity-fighter, antidiarrheal agent, antiviral agent, diuretic (caffeine), analgesic (caffeine), mild sedative (decaffeinated). In animals tea are potent blockers of various cancers. Tea drinkers appear to have less atherosclerosis (damaged, clogged arteries) and fewer strokes.

✔ **Tomatoes**

A major source of lycopene, an awesome antioxidant and anticancer agent that intervenes in devastating chain reactions of oxygen free radical molecules. Tomatoes are linked in particular to lower rates of pancreatic and cervical cancer.

✔ **Watermelon**

High amounts of lycopene and glutathione, anti-oxidant and anti-cancer compounds. Also mild antibacterial, anticoagulant activity.

Wheat

High-fiber whole wheat, and particularly wheat bran, rank as the world's greatest preventatives of constipation. The bran is potently anti-cancer. Remarkably, in humans, wheat bran can suppress polyps that can develop into colon cancer. In women wheat bran appears to antagonize breast cancer by diminishing supplies of estrogen. It is also antiparasitic. On the negative side, wheat ranks exceedingly high as a trigger of food intolerances and allergies.

✔ Wine

In moderation – a glass or two a day – benefits cardiovascular system. Both red and white wine boost heart-protecting HDL cholesterol. Red wine, in particular, seems to help ward off heart disease, blood clots and strokes because grape skins contain blood-thinning agents. (Grape skins are used in making red wine, but not white wine.) Boosts estrogen levels, which may accentuate wine's HDL-raising effects. Kills bacteria, inhibits viruses. May also discourage gallstones. An excess of wine, because of its alcohol, can cause heart, liver and brain damage.

✔ Yogurt

An ancient wonder food, strongly antibacterial and anticancer. A cup or two of yogurt a day boosts immune functioning and also spurs activity of natural killer cells that attack viruses and tumors. A daily cup of yogurt reduces colds and other upper respiratory infections in humans. Helps prevent and cure diarrhea as well as yeast infections in women. Helps fight bone problems, such as osteoporosis, because of high available calcium content. Acidophilus yogurt cultures neutralize cancer-causing agents in the intestinal tract. Plain old yogurt with L. bulgaricus and S. thermophilus cultures, both live and dead, blocked lung cancers in animals. Yogurt with live cultures is safe for people with lactose intolerance.

Source: Food – Your Miracle Medicine, copyright 1993 by Jean Carper and Harper Collins.

✔ My personal "Fit Happens" favorites.

The Muscle and Fitness Top 100
Bodybuilding Foods

Meat/Fish/Poultry*

	Calories (g)	Protein (g)	Carbs (g)	Fat (g)
Select top sirloin	180	30	0	6
Select top round	190	36	0	4
Select bottom round	171	29	0	5
Extra-lean ground beef	263	28	0	16
Skinless chicken breast	165	31	0	4
Skinless turkey breast	135	30	0	1
Pork tenderloin	164	28	0	5
Coho Salmon	184	27	0	7
Halibut	140	27	0	3
Canned light tuna	116	25	0	1
Scallops	88	17	2	1
Shrimp	99	21	0	1
Venison	158	30	0	3
Red snapper	128	26	0	2
Shark	130	21	0	5
Deli roast beef, 1 oz. Sliced	50	8	2	1
Deli ham	145	21	2	6
Lamb, choice, leg	191	28	0	8
Canadian-style bacon, grilled, 2 slices	86	11	1	4

Serving size is 3.5 oz., trimmed of all visible fat unless otherwise noted.

The Muscle and Fitness Top 100
Bodybuilding Foods

Grains/Breads/Pasta

	Calories (g)	Protein (g)	Carbs (g)	Fat (g)
Oatmeal, 1 c cooked	145	6	25	2
Whole-grain cereals, Total, ? c	110	3	24	1
Whole-wheat bread, 1 slice	69	3	13	1
Plain bagel, 1	195	7	38	1
English muffin	127	5	25	1
Whole-wheat pita, 1	170	6	35	2
Flour tortilla, 8-inch	145	4	25	3
Corn tortilla, 1	58	2	12	1
White rice, 1 c cooked	205	4	44	
Tr Brown rice, 1 c cooked	216	5	45	2
Wild rice, 1 c cooked	166	7	35	1
Couscous, 1 c cooked	176	6	36	Tr
Macaroni, 1 c cooked	197	7	40	1
Spaghetti, 1 c cooked	197	7	40	1
Bulgur, 1 c cooked	151	6	34	Tr
Wheat germ, 2 Tbsp.	50	4	6	1
Bran Muffin, Weight Watchers, 1	160	3	36	0
Sourdough bread, 1 slice	69	2	13	0
Whole-wheat crackers, 5	89	2	14	3
Whole-wheat pretzels, 1 oz.	103	3	23	0

The Muscle and Fitness Top 100
Bodybuilding Foods

Fruit

	Calories (g)	Protein (g)	Carbs (g)	Fat (g)
Cantaloupe, 1 c	55	1	13	Tr
Strawberries, 1 c	46	1	11	Tr
Blueberries, 1 c	81	1	20	Tr
Apple, 1	81	Tr	21	Tr
Orange, 1	64	1	16	Tr
Grapefruit, 1	37	Tr	9	0
Banana, 1	109	1	28	Tr
Kiwi, 1	46	Tr	11	Tr
Plum, 1	36	Tr	9	Tr
Peach, 1	42	Tr	11	Tr
Nectarine, 1	67	1	16	Tr
Apricot, 3	50	1	12	Tr
Grapes, 1 c seedless	114	1	28	1
Raisins, 1 c (not packed)	109	1	29	Tr
Pear, 1	98	Tr	25	Tr
Pineapple, 1 c	76	Tr	19	Tr
Orange juice, 1 c	112	2	26	Tr
Avocado, 1	77	1	3	8
Watermelon	49	1	11	1
Raspberries, 1 c	60	1	14	1

The Muscle and Fitness Top 100
Bodybuilding Foods

Vegetables

	Calories (g)	Protein (g)	Carbs (g)	Fat (g)
Broccoli florets, 1 c raw	20	2	4	Tr
Bell pepper (red, green), 1 c chopped	40	1	10	Tr
Onion, 1 c chopped	61	2	14	Tr
Tomato, 1 lg.	38	2	8	Tr
Asparagus, 4 spears	15	1	3	Tr
Collard greens, 1 c	11	Tr	3	Tr
Spinach, 1 c	7	1	1	Tr
Eggplant, 1 c cubed	11	Tr	3	Tr
Sweet potato, 1	117	2	28	Tr
Potato, 1 (approx. 7 oz.)	220	5	51	Tr
Carrot, 1	31	1	7	Tr
Green peas, 1 c	67	4	12	Tr
Corn, 1 c	89	3	21	1
Zucchini, ? c sliced	14	Tr	4	0
Garlic, 1 clove	4	Tr	1	0
Tomato juice, 1 c	46	2	11	Tr
Tomato sauce, 1 c	37	2	9	Tr
Romaine lettuce, 1 c shredded	9	1	1	Tr
Cucumber, 1 c	14	1	3	Tr
Mushrooms, 1 c	18	2	3	Tr
Cauliflower, 1 c	25	2	5	Tr
Green beans, 1 c	22	1	5	Tr
Artichoke, 1	60	4	13	Tr
Salsa, 1 c	29	1	6	Tr

The Muscle and Fitness Top 100
Bodybuilding Foods

Milk/Egg Products

	Calories (g)	Protein (g)	Carbs (g)	Fat (g)
Egg, large, 1 whole	75	6	1	5
Egg white, 1	17	4	Tr	0
Egg substitute, 1 c liquid	53	8	Tr	2
1% fat cottage cheese, 1 c	82	14	3	1
Low-fat cheddar cheese, 1 oz.	49	7	1	2
Plain nonfat yogurt, 8 oz.	127	13	17	Tr
Nonfat milk, 1 c	86	8	12	Tr
Raw firm tofu, 3.5 oz.	144	16	4	9
Swiss cheese, Healthy Choice, 1 slice	30	5	2	0

Legumes

Soybeans, 1 c cooked	149	14	9	8
Lentils, 1 c cooked	115	9	20	Tr
Black beans, 1 c cooked	114	8	20	1
Kidney beans, 1 c cooked	112	8	20	Tr
Baby lima beans, 1 c cooked	115	7	21	Tr

Nuts/Seeds

Peanut butter, 2 Tbsp.	190	8	6	16
Walnuts, 1 oz.	172	7	3	16
Flaxseeds, 3 Tbsp.	140	5	11	10
Peanuts, 1 oz. - dry roasted	166	7	6	14

Name, Date of Original Publication? - GCF

Nutritional Fat Loss Secrets

Nutrition is 24/7.

What you eat, and when, determines to a huge extent – how you look!

The 3,2,1 Nutritional Plan

According to some of the world's top exercise scientists (including Chris Aecto), cycling your carbohydrate consumption seems to be one of the best ways to get fit (i.e. ripped – a slang word in competitive fitness circles which means "very tight skin", which is 5% or 12% body fat or less for men and women respectively).

The 3,2,1 nutritional plan (not to be confused with the 3,2,1 priority training system mentioned earlier in this book) is one I use to lose the last few fat pounds around the lower abs and love handles.

The plan has you rotating your carbohydrate consumption every 3 days. Low carbs (about 50 grams a day) for three days (eating approximately 100-150 grams), then off, on again for two days, then off, and on again then back to three.

By cycling or rotating your "normal eating" carbohydrate days with a steady diet of 3,2,1 uncertainty **you will keep the body's "metabolic furnace" burning white hot!** This is because your body can never figure out when or what its next everyday food will be. There is too much positive and confusing change going on. Your body will burn high-octane because it doesn't know when or what it will get next.

Fit Happens for Seniors

One of my personal goals is to be the first person in our family to live to be 100 years old (Grandpa and Grandma Pierron are the current front-runners, living to be 96 and 92, respectively.)

To achieve such a goal, it's important to know and understand the many benefits of weight training and its positive effect on **longevity**.

• The American Heart association says a regular program of weight training may increase muscle strength and endurance, improve functioning of the heart and lungs, enhance glucose metabolism, reduce coronary disease risk factors and boost well-being.

• Experts are increasingly calling osteoporosis a pediatric disease with a geriatric outcome. The importance of exercise in skeletal health begins in youth: 30% of the skeleton can be formed during puberty, ages 9-14, which is a great time to instill the benefits of exercise. Bone deposits made during youth help sustain bone mass during the later years when bone loss occurs, particularly among post-menopausal women. **Resistance training that works bone and muscles against gravity 2-3 times a week provides major benefit without the risk of injury that can occur from many high-impact activities.**

• Cancer patients benefit from exercise, even when undergoing chemotherapy treatment or radiation therapy, according to a review of 24 studies. Regular physical activity reduces the risk of developing colon cancer common in obese people. Moderate physical activity is associated with a lower risk of colorectal cancer.

• Strength training may normalize resting blood pressure in 65-73-year-old men and women with high blood pressure.

• **Mayo Clinic physicians recommend exercise as a more proven and less costly strategy than injections of human growth hormone (hGH) in slowing and reversing the aging process.**

• Fit happens. Get in the game! Reverse the aging process naturally and set a goal to live to be 100 – in great health.

Source: Muscle & Fitness, December 2000

"Stay away from people who try to belittle your ambitions. Small people always do that. The really great people make you feel that you, too, can become great!"

- Mark Twain

America's Biggest Health Challenge

"If you're looking for a big opportunity,
seek out a big problem."

- Francis Pierron
Retired Dream Builder
P&L Construction

America's biggest health challenge at the moment is obesity.

Together, let's reverse the obesity trend, get fit by choice and continue to lead a fit lifestyle.

"It's never too late – in fiction or in life
– to revise."

-Nancy Thayer (author)

Revise your fitness commitment ... and begin again.

How to Train Intensely

"Be bold, be brief, be gone."
-Bonnie Griffin
SUNY 95 (94.7 FM)
Columbus, OH

(This is also an effective strategy for salespeople and an effective strategy for speaking to groups)

Genetics

Quit whining!

Your genetics (i.e. body type) are what your genetics are. Rejoice!

Granted, some are better than others at getting fit – but remember....
Your fitness potential is unlimited and controlled mostly by training,
nutrition and time (TNT).

Women and Strength Training

Myth #1: I won't be flexible if I lift weights.

Lifting weights will help you become more flexible. By following a proper strength training program, which involves going through a full range of motion each time, you will build flexibility.

Myth #2: I'm too old to lift weights.

You are never too old to help your muscles get fit.

Myth #3: I'm afraid I will look bulky and unfeminine.

Because women don't have enough of the male hormone testosterone, *they cannot bulk up like men*. Looking toned will not make you look "manly". Rather, you will be able to perform your everyday activities more efficiently. You will also be less likely to suffer injury if you are involved in a good strength training program.

Myth #4: Strength training isn't any fun.

Getting results is fun! As you build your strength, you will find that you actually enjoy working your muscles.

Steps for successful strength training.

Make it a priority to start training.
Consider using a personal trainer when you begin. He or she can help you find the routine that best meets your needs.

Chart your progress in an exercise journal so you can see how far you've come.

Take before and after photos every four months to maintain motivation.

Source: www.Healthresourcecenter.org

Don't know where to go to find a great trainer?

Email me direct at: **coachmike@drmbig.com** and I'll guide you through your initial steps via on-line training.

Short and Sweet

The TNT System is a high-intensity, short-duration training program.

The idea of abbreviated (short and intense) workouts has been around for 100 years or so. Bob Hoffman, Arthur Jones (the creator of Nautilus), Dorian Yates, Lee Labrada, Mike Mentzer, and many others have advocated and taught this advanced training knowledge.

It's easy to understand, then, why it works so well for the "natural" athlete. A few basic compound exercises that affect the whole body – so called "growth exercises" such as squats, deadlifts, bent-over rows, bench presses, chins and dips – would have the most direct and indirect growth effect on the body as a whole. These exercises work the largest muscles – and some of the smaller ones – very hard. You don't need a lot of sets on these growth exercises to cause the body to grow and get leaner.

Short and sweet wins the fat battle.

Unlimited Potential, Inc.

"Listen, my son, and be wise, and keep
your heart on the right path."

-Proverbs 23:19

Supersizing your natural potential is possible! Young adults, you do not
need drugs to succeed in sports or in life!

"Work hard (and smart), keep the faith
and be true to yourself."

-Joey and Jen's dad

Lose Two Pounds a Week – Guaranteed!

One pound = approximately 3,500 calories.

Seven days in one week.

3500 calories / 7 days = 500 calories a day.

Simply by lowering your calorie consumption (by 500 calories a day) and burning an extra 500 calories per day for one week, you will lose 2 pounds!

By both lowering consumption by 500 calories per day and exercising enough to burn another 500 calories per day you will lose approximately 1,000 (500 + 500 = 1,000) calories per day.

In one week, that will be 7,000 (7 x 1,000 = 7,000) calories lost. There's your two pounds. The beauty of the TNT system is you don't have to exercise every day in order to burn all those extra calories. In fact, you shouldn't. Properly followed, a couple times a week helps you burn calories 24/7!

My recommendation is to

not try to lose more than two pounds per week.

To lose more would imply under eating or overtraining.

The longer it takes to get off, the longer it will stay off!

Q. How many of you know someone that lost more than 20 pounds in a month on the Atkins Diet and has since gained all or most of it back?

A. I know quite a few.

X Factor Training

Many years ago, the Greek ideal was a "healthy mind and a healthy body." The Greeks glorified heroic strength and ideal human proportion. To them, a quality silhouette of a near flawless male physique consisted of stunning shoulders, full calves and tight abdominals – think Michelangelo and his "David" sculpture.

Fit Recommendation:
One day a week (for me, it's Wednesday) train only shoulders, calves and abs. Why? Shoulders, abs, and calves form a classic "X Factor" of the human body and look impressive to both sexes (both in clothes and out)!

Workout Words
March, 1990

While training for a natural physique competition, Mike Pierron, 27, needed something to keep him motivated on the days he didn't feel like working out. "I silk-screened the word 'Intensity' on a T-shirt," says Pierron, "and I wore it whenever I worked out."

Other gym members asked him where he had bought the shirt. Seizing an opportunity, Pierron printed T-shirts, muscle shirts, sweatshirts, and sweat pants with the words "Intensity" or "Desire" printed on them. The gym owner began selling the items at the club.

From these humble beginnings, Pierron began Motivational Selling, Inc., a Des Moines, Iowa-based company that offers seminars on motivation, selling and goal-setting. In addition, the company sells motivational apparel to local health clubs and athletic stores. Pierron hopes to eventually distribute the clothing to national sports apparel chains.

New Business Opportunities, 1990
(A division of Entrepreneur Magazine)

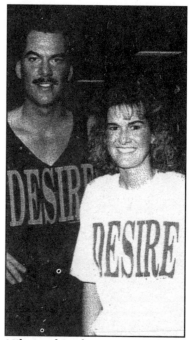

Mike and Linda Pierron hope their clothing will motivate sales.

Postscript

I believe that the **TNT System**, and the **"3,2,1 Priority System"** will produce positive results by helping people get into the best shape of their life.

My initial goal in writing this book was simple…to help reverse the current obesity trend in the United States.

A secondary goal has been to reach my fellow time-starved, Baby Boomers! There are 80 million of us in the U.S. between the ages of 37 and 55. If you've been searching for a "Fitness Cure" and getting results on a limited-cardio, high-intensity, 90 minute workout each week doesn't scare you…then results will come your way, too.

What does all this mean?

Step 1 has been (or will be) accomplished. You are finally **in control** over your most cherished possession – **your own body**. It's your health and your longevity.

What now? The sky's the limit. You decide.

But remember…

If it's meant to be, it's up to me!

I dare you…to Dream Big! And keep the momentum going.

God Bless!

"This is a must-read for everyone interested in improving their level of fitness. Mike's philosophy is simple, exciting, and it works!"
-*Jennifer Romagna*
2-Time Boston Marathon qualifier

"Mike, you are the BEST master of Ceremonies in Bodybuilding."
-*Stan McQuay*
2001 Superbody natural champion
www.stanmcquay.com

"We both loved the FIT HAPPENS CD! It was like you were in the room training with us."
-*Manny 35, and Jill 34, Johnson.*

"As a fellow HARDGAINER, your philosophy of be bold, be brief and be gone, (high-intensity-short duration) was perfect for me, and I'm sure millions of others. THANKS."
-*Jim Young, 32, Club West trainer*
@www.jimmy-fitness.com